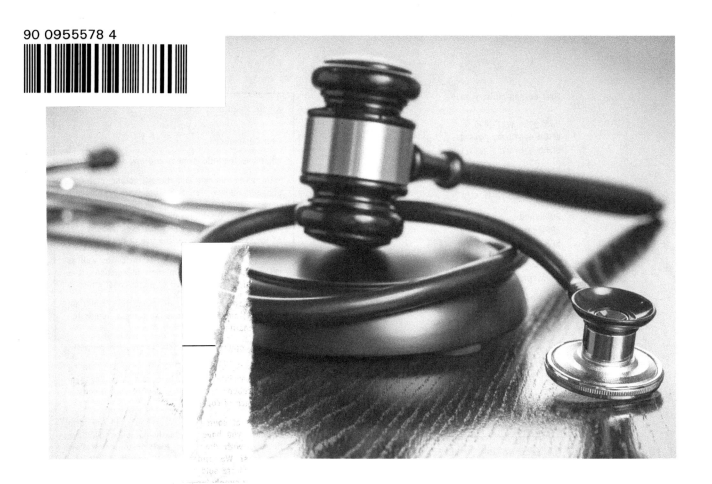

 sily Missed?:

Medico-legal pitfalls

Edited by
Professor Anthony Harnden &
Dr Richard Lehman

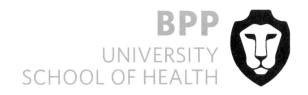

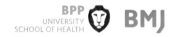

First edition January 2016

ISBN 9781 4727 3895 0
eISBN 9781 4727 3935 3
eISBN 9781 4727 3939 1

British Library Cataloguing-in-Publication Data
A catalogue record for this book is available
from the British Library

Published by
BPP Learning Media Ltd
BPP House, Aldine Place
London W12 8AA

www.bpp.com/health

Printed in the United Kingdom by
CPI Antony Rowe

Bumper's Farm,
Chippenham,
Wiltshire
SN14 6LH

Your learning materials, published by BPP Learning Media
Ltd, are printed on paper sourced from sustainable,
managed forests.

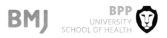

About the publisher

BPP Learning Media is dedicated to supporting aspiring professionals with top quality learning material. BPP Learning Media's commitment to success is shown by our record of quality, innovation and market leadership in paper-based and e-learning materials. BPP Learning Media's study materials are written by professionally-qualified specialists who know from personal experience the importance of top quality materials for success.

About The BMJ

The BMJ (formerly the British Medical Journal) in print has a long history and has been published without interruption since 1840. The BMJ's vision is to be the world's most influential and widely read medical journal. Our mission is to lead the debate on health and to engage, inform, and stimulate doctors, researchers, and other health professionals in ways that will improve outcomes for patients. We aim to help doctors to make better decisions. BMJ, the company, advances healthcare worldwide by sharing knowledge and expertise to improve experiences, outcomes and value.

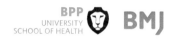

Contents

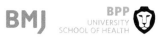

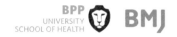

About the editors

Professor Anthony Harnden is an academic general practitioner at the University of Oxford who has worked five clinical sessions as a partner in general practice in Wheatley, Oxfordshire for more than 25 years. He has published original research papers in general practice related topics, with a focus on children. Professor Harnden is a Deputy Chairman of the Joint Committee of Vaccination and Immunisation (JCVI) and has been responsible for advising the UK government on vaccine policy since 2006. He was the primary care lead for the UK Confidential Enquiry into Child Deaths (2004-8), chaired a group to write a national Royal College of General Practitioners Child Health Strategy (2010-15) and developed the successful series 'Easily Missed?' in The BMJ (2009-).

Dr Richard Lehman is Senior Advisory Fellow in General Practice at the UK Cochrane Centre. He was a full-time general practitioner in Banbury for 32 years. For the last 17 years he has also written a weekly summary of the principal medical journals which is posted on The BMJ website. After retirement from UK general practice in 2010 he has worked on studies of the patient experience, and has spent a year at Yale working with the Yale University Open Data Access (YODA) project and remains a consultant to the group. His main interest is in ways to develop better informed dialogue with patients and he is on the steering committees of the NICE shared decision making initiative and Academy of Medical Royal Colleges Choosing Wisely group.

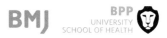

Foreword

"To err is human". So said Alexander Pope. And nowhere is it more true than in medicine. The general practitioner in his encounters with patients is only too aware of the possibility of making mistakes since he, above all, has to tolerate a high measure of diagnostic uncertainty and must make clinical judgements in a short space of time.

Failure to diagnose certain conditions can have disastrous consequences both for the patient and for the doctor. For the patient it can mean delay and frustration and a loss of trust in the clinician; at worst, it can result in permanent disability and even death. For the doctor it may result in a complaint, sometimes lengthy litigation and even a referral to the General Medical Council. Anything that can be done to alert the clinician to possible pitfalls is worthwhile; hence this collection of articles.

Included are conditions that are easily missed, even in skilled hands. The collection is not meant to be comprehensive, nor is it necessarily a reflection of those conditions that frequently result in large pay-outs for the claimant, but it nevertheless contains salutary lessons for all engaged in making early diagnoses.

Take, for example, sub-dural haematoma in the elderly. As is pointed out in the article, only half of those diagnosed give a history of direct trauma to the head or of a fall involving the head. There can be a long delay between the trauma itself and the onset of symptoms, and those symptoms can easily be misinterpreted. They can mimic alcohol excess, a change in someone's personality or even dementia. The doctor needs to have a high index of suspicion in patients giving a recent history of falls or who exhibit behavioural or cognitive changes. It matters because early surgical intervention can reverse the deterioration whilst delay can result in permanent neurological deficit and death.

Other conditions mentioned, such as phaeochromocytoma, are much less common and therefore rarely considered in any differential diagnosis. One can go a lifetime and not see a case. A phaeo. is easily missed because the signs and symptoms vary and can easily be confused with other much more common conditions. Nevertheless it is important not to miss the diagnosis since it carries a high morbidity and mortality. Raising awareness even in this relatively rare condition can pay huge dividends.

The examples listed in the book are wide ranging, some common, some uncommon, but all provide a challenge to the busy G.P. In modern day practice pressure of time and lack of follow-up can lead to delay in diagnosis and, in turn, to litigation where there has been perceived negligence.

Of course, a fresh pair of eyes can uncover a pitfall, though more usually the written comments of the last doctor are taken at face value and further enquiry is deemed unnecessary. Having an awareness of the potential significance of certain symptoms and relying on intuition in certain circumstances where the pattern of symptoms is unusual can be of assistance. So too can reading these articles written by experts in the field. I thoroughly recommend them to you.

Dr Peter Williams

President and Chairman of the Medical Defence Union

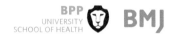

Introduction to Easily Missed series

Patients consult doctors with the expectation of an accurate diagnosis and advice on treatment. But in primary care, patients often present with undifferentiated symptoms without an immediately apparent diagnosis. For most conditions this doesn't matter because the symptoms either resolve or become worse in such a way that the patient returns before any harm is done. In consultations, general practitioners work by using the probability that the collection of presenting symptoms reflects a specific diagnosis. A combination of knowledge, clinical experience, and sound judgment ensures that they usually get it right.

The BMJ series "Easily Missed?" has raised awareness among general practitioners of conditions that are under-recognised in primary care at first presentation. The series has included a wide range of conditions, including some that are common but under-diagnosed and others that are uncommon but so serious that they need to be thought of whenever there is any possibility of their existence.

The articles are short and focused on diagnosis at presentation rather than treatment. The conditions described fulfil four key criteria. Firstly, there is evidence that the condition is commoner than most general practitioners realise or is often missed at first presentation. Secondly, the condition is sufficiently common that the average full time general practitioner in the UK will encounter it at least once a year, or else be so serious that delayed diagnosis is likely to worsen prognosis substantially. Thirdly, the condition has easily defined diagnostic features or diagnostic tests with known predictive characteristics. Fourthly, and most importantly, timely recognition will benefit the patient.

Judging from online access, the series has proved popular amongst readers of The BMJ. We hope that many patients have received early and insightful diagnoses as a result. The series would not have been possible without the dedication, hard work and wisdom of our in house editor, Dr Mabel Chew. She has been a delight to work with and we are very grateful for all her efforts.

Osler said "Medicine is a science of uncertainty and an art of probability." Although uncertainty will always be with us in primary care, the series might teach us more about the art of probability.

Anthony Harnden and Richard Lehman

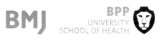

Pulmonary embolism

Guy Meyer, MD[1] [2] [3], Pierre-Marie Roy, MD PhD[4],
Serge Gilberg, MD[1], Arnaud Perrier, MD[5]

[1]Université Paris Descartes, Paris, France

[2]Assistance Publique Hôpitaux de Paris, Hôpital Européen Georges Pompidou, Service de Pneumologie et Soins Intensifs, Paris, France

[3]INSERM Unité 765, Paris, France

[4]Université d'Angers, IFR 132 et Centre Hospitalier Universitaire, Service d'accueil et traitement des urgences, Angers, France

[5]Division of General Internal Medicine, Geneva University Hospital, Switzerland

Correspondence to: Dr G Meyer, Service de Pneumologie, Hopital Europeen Georges Pompidou, 20 rue Leblanc, 75015 Paris, France, guy.meyer@egp.aphp.fr

Cite this as: BMJ 2010;340:C1421

DOI: 10.1136/bmj.c1421

www.bmj.com/content/340/bmj.c1421

Complete occlusion of a peripheral pulmonary artery usually results in a pulmonary infarction with pleuritic chest pain and haemoptysis. When the blood clot is lodged in more proximal pulmonary arteries and is not occlusive, pulmonary infarction does not occur and pulmonary embolism might present as isolated dyspnoea. Massive pulmonary embolism is caused by large bilateral proximal clots resulting in haemodynamic collapse.[1]

Why is it missed?

The classic triad of pleuritic chest pain, dyspnoea, and haemoptysis occurs in less than 10% of patients, but the most common symptoms (dyspnoea, chest pain) are non-specific. In 40% of cases, major thromboembolic risk factors are absent. Clinical signs of deep vein thrombosis are observed in only 15% of patients and haemoptysis in only 4.5-11% of cases.[1] [5] Pulmonary infarction with fever may mimic pneumonia. Chest pain reproducible on palpation also does not rule out pulmonary embolism.[6] In addition, abnormalities in chest radiographs or electrocardiograms are non-specific; sinus tachycardia is the most common electrocardiogram abnormality whereas right heart strain is observed only in severe cases. Arterial partial pressure of oxygen and the alveolar-arterial oxygen gradient are normal in 20% of patients; hypoxaemia with hypocapnia is the most common abnormality in blood gas pressures, but is non-specific.[1] Symptoms and initial test findings can also be ascribed to underlying disease such as heart failure or chronic lung disease.[7]

Why does it matter?

Without adequate treatment, pulmonary embolism recurs in 30-50% of cases, with a case fatality rate of between 10-45%.[8] Non-diagnosed cases therefore have a high risk of recurrence and death.

How is it diagnosed?

Consider a diagnosis of pulmonary embolism in patients with:

- Dyspnoea, pleuritic chest pain, and haemoptysis
- Any chest symptoms and clinical features suggesting deep vein thrombosis
- Dyspnoea or chest pain, and a major risk factor for pulmonary embolism (table)
- Unexplained dyspnoea, chest pain, or mild haemoptysis, whether or not they have minor risk factors for pulmonary embolism.

Once the diagnosis is suspected, conduct a clinical or pre-test probability assessment based on risk factors and clinical features, as post-test probability depends on test characteristics and pre-test probability. The assessment can be done either by implicit clinical judgment or by using a validated prediction rule such as the Geneva or Wells scores (table). These

---

KEY POINTS

- Suspect pulmonary embolism in cases of unexplained dyspnoea or chest pain, or both, even in the absence of obvious risk or triggering factors
- Clinical probability assessment is the cornerstone of all validated diagnostic strategies
- Always conduct objective tests to confirm or exclude suspected pulmonary embolism. Most patients diagnosed and treated according to guidelines have an uneventful outcome. On the other hand, unrecognised and untreated pulmonary embolism carries a 50% risk of recurrence and a 25% risk of death

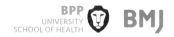

Table 1 Geneva revised score			Wells score	
Variables	Points	Variables		Points
Predisposing factors				
Age >65 years	1	–		–
Previous venous thromboembolism	3	Previous DVT or PE		1.5
Surgery or fracture <1 month	2	Recent surgery or immobilisation		1.5
Active malignancy	2	Cancer		1
Symptoms				
Unilateral lower limb pain	3	–		–
Haemoptysis	2	Haemoptysis		1
Clinical signs				
Heart rate 75-94 bpm	3	–		–
Heart rate ≥95 bpm	5	Heart rate >100 beats/min		1.5
Unilateral lower limb oedema and pain	4	Clinical signs of DVT		3
–	–	Alternative diagnosis less likely than PE		3
Clinical probability				
Low	0-3	Low		0-1
Intermediate	4-10	Intermediate		2-6
High	≥11	High		≥7

DVT=deep vein thrombosis, PE=pulmonary embolism.

rules have a fair accuracy in large prospective series of patients with suspected pulmonary embolism: prevalence of pulmonary embolism is about 10% in patients with a low clinical probability, 30% in those with a moderate clinical probability, and 65% in those with a high clinical probability.[9] [10]

Investigations

- Plasma D-dimer measurement is the next step for most outpatients. D-dimer levels are raised in many situations and a positive test result is non-specific. However, based on a negative likelihood ratio of 0.08, a negative result for a quantitative, enzyme linked immunosorbent assay (ELISA) D-dimer test excludes pulmonary embolism and the need for further testing in about 30% of patients, provided that the clinical probability is low or moderate.[11] Quantitative latex based and whole blood qualitative D-dimer assays have a negative likelihood ratio of 0.20 to 0.30 and allow exclusion of pulmonary embolism only in patients with a low probability.[11] In patients with a high clinical probability, no D-dimer test is sensitive enough to rule out pulmonary embolism.

- Refer patients with a positive D-dimer test for multidetector spiral computed tomography. This procedure confirms pulmonary embolism when an intraluminal defect is seen in several subsegmental arteries or in a more proximal pulmonary artery (figure).[12] A ventilation and perfusion lung scan may be selected when multidetector spiral computed tomography is contraindicated (renal failure, allergy to contrast medium) but yields a high rate of inconclusive results. Finally, compression ultrasonography of the leg veins showing a proximal deep vein thrombosis in a patient with thoracic symptoms allows confirmation of pulmonary embolism without further testing, but has a low diagnostic yield, except in patients with clinical symptoms of deep vein thrombosis.[9] [11]

- Excluding pulmonary embolism on inappropriate criteria, for example, low D-dimer reading in a patient with a high clinical probability or a low probability lung scan in a patient with a high clinical probability, exposes patients to an increase risk of it recurring and death.[7]

How is it managed?

In patients with a high clinical probability, start anticoagulant treatment before objective confirmation of the disease. Low molecular weight heparin and fondaparinux are the first line options but are contraindicated in patients with severe renal insufficiency. In these patients, unfractionated heparin is still used for initial treatment.[13] Start vitamin K antagonists on the first day and give for at least three months.[13]

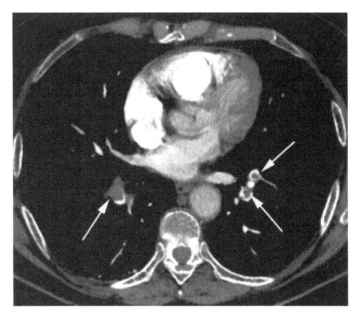

Fig 1 Multidetector spiral computed tomogram showing bilateral filling defects [arrowed] in the pulmonary artery

---

CASE SCENARIO

A non-smoking, previously well woman in her 70s complained of recent onset of dyspnoea. She had no cardiovascular or thromboembolic risk factors and clinical examination was normal apart from a heart rate of 96 beats per minute. With no clear explanation for the symptoms, her general practitioner applied a decision rule (table) to evaluate the clinical probability of pulmonary embolism. The result was intermediate, prompting him to request a D-dimer level, which was raised. He referred the patient to hospital, where pulmonary embolism was confirmed on computed tomography.

HOW COMMON IS IT?

- The incidence of diagnosed pulmonary embolism increases with age

- The annual rate is about 1 in 10 000 in individuals below 40 years of age and can reach 1 in 100 in patients over 80 years[2] [3]

- According to autopsy studies, the disease is clinically suspected in less than half of fatal cases, so the real incidence is probably underestimated[4]

- However, most episodes of pulmonary embolism carry a low mortality risk (about 1%) when properly diagnosed and treated

- Massive pulmonary embolism represents only 5% of all cases of pulmonary embolism and is fatal in about 40% of patients[1]

Contributors: All authors contributed equally to the design and drafting and approved the final version of the submitted article. All authors are guarantors.

Competing interests: None declared.

Provenance and peer review: Not commissioned; externally peer reviewed.

Patient consent not required (patient anonymised, dead, or hypothetical).

1 Torbicki A, Perrier A, Konstantinides S, Agnelli G, Galiè N, Pruszczyk P, et al. Guidelines on the diagnosis and management of acute pulmonary embolism: the Task Force for the Diagnosis and Management of Acute Pulmonary Embolism of the European Society of Cardiology (ESC). *Eur Heart J* 2008;29:2276-315.

2 Oger E. Incidence of venous thromboembolism: a community-based study in western France. EPI-GETBP Study Group. Groupe d'Etude de la Thrombose de Bretagne Occidentale. *Thromb Haemost* 2000;83:657-60.

3 Nordström M, Lindblad B. Autopsy-verified venous thromboembolism within a defined urban population-the city of Malmo, Sweden. *APMIS* 1998;106:378-84.

4 Pineda LA, Hathwar VS, Grant BJ. Clinical suspicion of fatal pulmonary embolism. *Chest* 2001;120:791-5.

5 Le Gal G, Righini M, Roy PM, Sanchez O, Aujesky D, Bounameaux H, et al. Prediction of pulmonary embolism in the emergency department: the revised Geneva score. *Ann Intern Med* 2006;144:165-71.

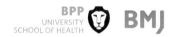

6   Le Gal G, Testuz A, Righini M, Bounameaux H, Perrier A. Reproduction of chest pain by palpation: diagnostic accuracy in suspected pulmonary embolism. *BMJ* 2005;330:452-3.

7   Roy PM, Meyer G, Vielle B, Le Gall C, Verschuren F, Carpentier F, et al. Appropriateness of diagnostic management and outcomes of suspected pulmonary embolism. *Ann Intern Med* 2006;144:157-64.

8   Meyer G, Planquette B, Sanchez O. Long-term outcome of pulmonary embolism. *Curr Opin Hematol* 2008;15:499-503.

9   Righini M, Le Gal G, Aujesky D, Roy PM, Sanchez O, Verschuren F, et al. Diagnosis of pulmonary embolism by multidetector CT alone or combined with venous ultrasonography of the leg: a randomised non-inferiority trial. *Lancet* 2008;371:1343-52.

10 Van Belle A, Büller HR, Huisman MV, Huisman PM, Kaasjager K, Kamphuisen PW, et al. Effectiveness of managing suspected pulmonary embolism using an algorithm combining clinical probability, D-dimer testing, and computed tomography. *JAMA* 2006;295:172-9.

11 Roy PM, Colombet I, Durieux P, Chatellier G, Sors H, Meyer G. Systematic review and meta-analysis of strategies for the diagnosis of suspected pulmonary embolism. *BMJ* 2005;331:259.

12 Stein PD, Fowler SE, Goodman LR, Gottschalk A, Hales CA, Hull RD, et al. Multidetector computed tomography for acute pulmonary embolism. *N Engl J Med* 2006;354:2317-27.

13 Kearon C, Kahn SR, Agnelli G, Goldhaber S, Raskob GE, Comerota AJ. Antithrombotic therapy for venous thromboembolic disease: American College of Chest Physicians Evidence-Based Clinical Practice Guidelines (8th Edition). *Chest* 2008;133:454S-5S.

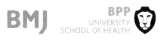
Acute leg ischaemia

Stephen Brearley, consultant surgeon

Whipps Cross University
Hospital, London E11
1NR, UK

vascusurg@btconnect.
com

Cite this as: BMJ
2013;346:f2681

DOI: 10.1136/bmj.f2681

www.bmj.com/
content/346/bmj.f2681

A 55 year old man consulted his general practitioner complaining of persistent pain in his left leg for three days and a numb feeling in the foot. He was taking treatment for hypertension, had a history of low back pain, and was a smoker of 20 cigarettes a day. His foot looked normal, but sensation seemed mildly reduced. The general practitioner noted a weak dorsalis pedis pulse. A diagnosis of sciatica was made, diclofenac was prescribed, and the patient was invited to return a week later if no better. Six days later he presented to a local emergency department because of intolerable pain and was found to have a profoundly ischaemic left leg necessitating an above knee amputation.

Missed diagnoses of acute leg ischaemia, as in the case above, are common.[1][2] An analysis of data held by the NHS Litigation Authority (NHSLA), the Medical Defence Union (MDU), and the Medical Protection Society (MPS) identified 224 cases of acute leg ischaemia leading to limb loss over a 10 year period,[1] in all of which litigation had been initiated. Fifty one cases in which there had been delay in detecting and treating acute limb ischaemia were reported to the National Reporting and Learning System (NRLS) between 2003 and 2010.[2] I have written almost 30 medicolegal reports on cases in which there were allegations—usually against general practitioners or casualty officers—of a negligent delay in diagnosing acute leg ischaemia, often resulting in the avoidable loss of a limb.

What is acute leg ischaemia?

Leg ischaemia results from thrombotic, embolic, or traumatic arterial occlusion. It is considered to be acute if the symptoms and signs have developed over less than two weeks.[3][4] The term "acute ischaemia" does not of itself imply severe ischaemia, but the survival of an acutely ischaemic limb is often in immediate jeopardy.[2] The hallmarks of acute ischaemia that is limb threatening are reduced muscular power and reduced sensation in the limb.

How common is it?

In a 1996 questionnaire survey of members of the Vascular Surgical Society of Great Britain and Ireland, 86 out of 182 hospitals reported 539 episodes of acute lower limb ischaemia in a three month period.[4] In this study, acute lower limb ischaemia was defined as "a previously stable limb with sudden deterioration in the arterial supply for less than two weeks." In another study, an incidence as high as one per 7000 per annum has been quoted.[5] Medicolegal data[1] show that over 20 legal actions are initiated each year in the UK in relation to acute leg ischaemia, with delay in diagnosis or treatment figuring in 73% of the claims.

Why is it missed?

In the cases reported to the NRLS, the National Patient Safety Agency stated that causes of delay in detecting and treating acute limb ischaemia included diagnostic errors (such as misdiagnosis as a Baker's cyst or disc problem, as in the case scenario), acute limb ischaemia not being recognised as a surgical emergency, and apparently inconsistent clinical diagnosis and assessment. My own clinical and medicolegal experience indicates that there is often a failure to consider a diagnosis of acute leg ischaemia at all, especially if the patient is under 60 years old (as in the case scenario). By no means all patients with acute leg ischaemia have risk factors (such as atrial fibrillation, a history of smoking, or diabetes). It should therefore be considered in the differential diagnosis of all patients presenting with leg pain of sudden onset, irrespective of age and risk factors, and all such patients should undergo an assessment of the circulation to the limb.

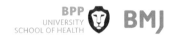

The extent to which acutely ischaemic legs are pale (or discoloured) or cold or exhibit diminished power or sensation is variable, and subtle changes can be missed (as in the case above) if the examination is cursory. An error encountered in almost all cases of missed acute leg ischaemia, however, is that one or more doctors have purported to feel pulses that could not possibly have been present. Pulse palpation is an unreliable physical sign, with false positive palpation occurring in 14% of observations carried out by non-specialists.[6] A "weak" or "faint" ankle pulse, or one which the doctor "thinks" he or she can feel, is probably not present at all (as in the case history above). A simple rule will protect against this common error: "If you can feel a pulse you can count it; if you cannot count it, you are not feeling it."

Why does it matter?

Delay in diagnosis or referral was the sole or the principal cause of amputation in 59% of the patients identified from medicolegal data.[1] The interval between the onset of symptoms and irretrievable damage to the leg is variable but may be as little as six hours.[2 7] Acute leg ischaemia is associated with an amputation rate of 13% and a mortality of 10%.[8] Both are increased by delay in diagnosis and treatment.[8]

How is it diagnosed?

Acute leg ischaemia can only be diagnosed if it is included in the differential diagnosis of leg pain of recent onset. It should be considered in patients of all ages. Although usually encountered in patients over 60 years old, rare disorders (such as popliteal entrapment syndrome, cystic adventitial disease, and thrombophilias) may occasionally lead to its development in much younger individuals.

In all patients presenting with leg pain of sudden onset, look for the symptoms and signs of limb threatening ischaemia as characterised by the "six Ps" (see box). The patient will always have persistent pain and the ankle pulses will always be absent. The other Ps may or may not be present, depending on severity, and if present may be subtle (as in the case above). The presence or absence of risk factors for peripheral arterial disease is of limited usefulness. Limb threatening ischaemia may develop in individuals who have no known risk factors and are well under the age of 60.

The presence of acute leg ischaemia can be quickly, simply, and reliably confirmed or ruled out by measuring the ankle blood pressure with a pocket Doppler machine and a blood pressure cuff.[9] The absence of Doppler signals indicates a threatened limb, and the patient requires emergency referral to a vascular centre. Doppler assessment can be quickly learnt, is reproducible, and is easier than many other procedures routinely carried out in primary care (such as funduscopy). Pocket Doppler machines are cheap (approximately £300).

How is it managed?

If a patient has leg pain of recent onset and has impalpable pulses, immediate referral to a vascular surgical unit is mandatory. The management undertaken there will depend on the immediacy of the threat to the survival of the limb. The key clinical indicators of this are

---

LEG ISCHAEMIA—THE "6 PS"

- *Pain*—Always present, persistent
- *Pallor* or cyanosis or mottling*
- *Perishing* with cold (poikilothermia)*
- *Pulselessness*—Always present. Can you count it?
- *Paraesthesia* or reduced sensation or numbness*
- *Paralysis* or reduced power*

*May be subtle. Compare left and right legs

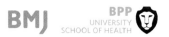

the presence and severity of reduced muscular power and reduced sensation. Depending on the urgency of the situation, the vascular unit may carry out imaging studies of the arteries supplying blood to the leg (duplex ultrasound, magnetic resonance angiography, computed tomographic angiography or intra-arterial angiography) as a basis for planning treatment. The options for treatment comprise endovascular procedures (angioplasty, thrombectomy, and intra-arterial thrombolysis) and surgery (embolectomy and bypass).[7] In an immediately threatened limb, emergency surgery will be required. Regrettably, some patients present with limbs that are already dead (profound paralysis and numbness, fixed mottling of the skin). In this situation revascularisation may be not merely futile but harmful, and primary amputation is necessary.[8]

Contributors: The article's content was developed in discussion with J Murray Longmore, and the first draft was revised in the light of comments from Longmore.

Competing interests: I have read and understood the BMJ Group policy on declaration of interests and have no relevant interests to declare.

Provenance and peer review: Commissioned; externally peer reviewed.

Patient consent: Patient consent not required (patient anonymised, dead, or hypothetical).

1   Shearman A, Shearman C. Failure to diagnose acute limb ischaemia (ALI); an avoidable cause of limb loss. Association of Surgeons of Great Britain and Ireland, 2012 International Surgical Congress. In: www.asgbi.org.uk/liverpool2012/pdfs/oral_shortpapers/Vascular_I.pdf abstract 0812.

2   National Patient Safety Agency. Early detection and treatment of acute limb ischaemia. Signal. 2011. www.nrls.npsa.nhs.uk/resources/?EntryId45=130172.

3   Creager MA, Kaufman JA, Conte MS. Acute limb ischaemia. N Engl J Med 2012;366:2198-206.

4   Campbell WB, Ridler BMF, Szymanska TH. Current management of acute leg ischaemia: results of an audit by the Vascular Surgical Society of Great Britain and Ireland. Br J Surg 1998;85:1498-503.

5   Trummer G, Brehm K, Siepe M, Heilmann C, Schlensak C, Beyersdorf F. The management of acute limb ischemia. Minerva Chir 2010;65:319-28.

6   Brearley S, Shearman CP, Simms MH. Peripheral pulse palpation: an unreliable physical sign. Ann Roy Coll Surg Engl 1992;74:169-71.

7   Earnshaw JJ. Acute ischaemia: evaluation and decision making. In: Cronenwett JL, Johnston KW, eds. Rutherford's vascular surgery. 7th ed. Saunders Elsevier, 2010:2389-98.

8   Henke P. Contemporary management of acute limb ischaemia: factors associated with amputation and in-hospital mortality. Semin Vasc Surg 2009;22:34-40.

9   National Institute for Health and Clinical Excellence. Lower limb peripheral arterial disease: diagnosis and management. (Clinical guideline 147.) 2012. http://guidance.nice.org.uk/CG147.

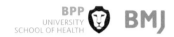

Ectopic pregnancy

Sheikha Al-Jabri, fellow of minimally invasive gynaecology,
Michael Malus, associate professor, department of family medicine,
Togas Tulandi, professor of obstetrics and gynaecology,
Milton Leong, chair in reproductive medicine

McGill University, Montreal, QC, Canada H3A 1A1

Correspondence to: S Al-Jabri s_umreem@hotmail.com

Cite this as: BMJ 2010;341:c3770

DOI: 10.1136/bmj.c3770

www.bmj.com/content/341/bmj.c3770

In women of reproductive age, ruling out ectopic pregnancy is mandatory as it is still the leading cause of death in the first trimester of pregnancy. This needs a high index of suspicion and an early pregnancy test. A negative test result excludes ectopic pregnancy, and a positive result demands further clinical, biochemical, and ultrasound examination to exclude or confirm ectopic pregnancy. The possibility of medical treatment for ectopic pregnancy makes early diagnosis even more important.

How common is it?

The estimated incidence of ectopic pregnancy in the United Kingdom is 11.1 per 1000 reported pregnancies.[1] However, some of these cases could be misdiagnosed. A retrospective study estimated that 12% of ectopic pregnancies were missed at initial presentation.[2] In a prospective consecutive case series among women with ectopic pregnancy who attended the emergency department, 45% were discharged with a wrong diagnosis.[3]

Why is it missed?

In a review of 31 cases of missed ectopic pregnancy, several important factors contributing to misdiagnosis were identified:[2]

- Failure to consider a possible pregnancy
- Failure to place importance on known risk factors
- Failure to consider an ectopic pregnancy in the differential diagnosis
- Failure to correlate serum concentration of ß human chorionic gonadotropin (ß hCG) with results of transvaginal ultrasound
- Failure to arrange suitable follow-up.

Why does this matter?

Early diagnosis reduces morbidity and mortality, as most ectopic pregnancies can now be treated safely and effectively with methotrexate.[4] In most cases, surgery is no longer needed. Late diagnosis could lead to tubal rupture and haemoperitoneum, requiring emergency surgery and removal of the fallopian tube.[5]

How is it diagnosed?

Clinical features

Traditionally, the diagnosis of ectopic pregnancy is made by history of pelvic pain associated with amenorrhea, and a positive pregnancy test with or without vaginal bleeding. Risk

---

KEY POINTS FOR DIAGNOSIS

- Suspect ectopic pregnancy in women of reproductive age who have abdominal pain and amenorrhea with or without vaginal bleeding
- Consider risk factors for ectopic pregnancy: history of tubal ectopic pregnancy, pelvic inflammatory disease, previous tubal surgery, fertility treatment, smoking, and multiple sexual partners
- Positive results on urine or serum hCG testing
- Perform transvaginal ultrasound and correlate with serum ß hCG concentrations

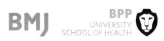

factors include history of tubal ectopic pregnancy, pelvic inflammatory disease, previous tubal surgery, fertility treatment, smoking, and multiple sexual partners.

Studies on predictive value of history and physical examination in patients with suspected ectopic pregnancy showed no constellation of findings that confirm or exclude the diagnosis with a high degree of reliability.[6][7] Definitive diagnosis at an early stage of pregnancy usually requires a combination of transvaginal ultrasound examination and measurement of human chorionic gonadotrophin (hCG).

Investigations

A commercial urine pregnancy test can be used as a screening test in primary care. The minimal detectable levels of urinary hCG vary from 25 IU/l to 50 IU/l. Thus if clinical features are suspicious and the urine test is positive, referral for more definitive diagnosis would be warranted.

If the test for serum ß hCG is readily available, it may help diagnosis. An intrauterine gestational sac is typically visible when serum ß hCG concentration is beyond the discriminatory zone (1500 IU/l) at 5 weeks' gestation. If the concentration is higher than this level and ultrasound does not show an intrauterine pregnancy but shows a complex adnexal mass, an extrauterine pregnancy is almost certain. An ectopic pregnancy can also be suspected if the serum hCG concentration is not increasing or if it plateaus. If feasible, a serum ß hCG test showing <1500 IU/l should be repeated in three days to follow the rate of rise; if hCG concentration does not double over 72 hours, then the pregnancy is abnormal (an ectopic gestation or failed intrauterine pregnancy). If it is not possible to repeat the hCG measurement, primary care practitioners could refer the patient to the gynaecologist for more definitive diagnosis.

In primary care, transvaginal ultrasound may not be readily available and transabdominal ultrasound is considered a useful screening test for early pregnancy complications, with a sensitivity of 80% and specificity of 78%.[8] Finding an intrauterine gestation on abdominal scan effectively excludes the possibility of an ectopic pregnancy. However, ultrasound diagnosis should be made by visualising an adnexal mass rather than the absence of intrauterine sac only. For more definitive diagnosis, the sensitivity of transvaginal ultrasound to diagnose tubal ectopic pregnancy is 90.9% and the specificity is 99.9%.[8]

Progesterone concentration is higher in viable intrauterine pregnancies than in ectopic and non-viable intrauterine pregnancies, but this test is unhelpful in diagnosis as it does not distinguish ectopic pregnancies from failed intrauterine pregnancies.[9]

How is it managed?

The optimal candidates for medical treatment with methotrexate are haemodynamically stable patients, willing and able to comply with follow-up, who have a serum ß hCG concentration of ≤5000 IU/l and no fetal cardiac activity. The overall success rate of methotrexate treatment in properly selected women is about 90%.[4]

Surgical treatment is indicated in some situations: haemodynamic instability, impending tubal rupture, contraindications to methotrexate, coexisting intrauterine pregnancy (heterotopic pregnancy), not able or willing to comply with follow-up after treatment, lack of timely access to a medical institution for management of tubal rupture, and failed medical treatment.

CASE SCENARIO

A 33 year-old woman presented to the emergency department with a five day history of low abdominal pain. Her last menstrual period was five weeks before; she said she was using progesterone-only pills for contraception and had a history of *Chlamydia* infection, so a pregnancy test was not done. She was diagnosed with pelvic inflammatory disease and prescribed antibiotics. She returned to the emergency department two days later with worsening abdominal pain, hypotension, and tachycardia. An urgent pregnancy test and ultrasonography led to the diagnosis of a tubal ectopic pregnancy.

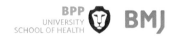

All authors contributed to planning and conduct; SA and TT contributed to reporting and writing the manuscript. TT is guarantor.

Competing interests: All authors have completed the unified competing interest form at www.icmje. org/coi_disclosure.pdf (available on request from the corresponding author) and declare no support from any organisation for the submitted work; no financial relationships with any organisation that might have an interest in the submitted work in the previous three years; and no other relationships or activities that could appear to have influenced the submitted work.

Provenance and peer review: Commissioned; externally peer reviewed.

1   Lewis G. Confidential Enquiry into Maternal and Child Health (CEMACH). Saving mothers' lives: reviewing maternal deaths to make motherhood safer—2003-2005. The seventh report on confidential enquiries into maternal deaths in the United Kingdom. London: CEMACH, 2007:92-3.
2   Robson SJ, O'Shea RT. Undiagnosed ectopic pregnancy: a retrospective analysis of 31'missed'ectopic pregnancies at a teaching hospital. *Aust N Z J Obstet Gynaecol* 1996;36:182-5.
3   Stovall T, Kellerman A, Ling F, Buster J. Emergency department diagnosis of ectopic pregnancy. *Ann Emerg Med* 1990;19:1098-103.
4   Lipscomb G, McCord M, Stovall T, Huff G, Portera S, Ling F. Predictors of success of methotrexate treatment in women with tubal ectopic pregnancies. *N Engl J Med* 1999;341:1974.
5   Job-Spira N, Fernandez H, Bouyer J, Pouly J, Germain E, Coste J. Ruptured tubal ectopic pregnancy: Risk factors and reproductive outcome: results of a population-based study in France. *Am J Obstet Gynecol* 1999;180:938-44.
6   Dart R, Kaplan B, Varaklis K. Predictive value of history and physical examination in patients with suspected ectopic pregnancy. *Ann Emerg Med* 1999;33(3):283-90.
7   Buckley R, King K, Disney J, Gorman J, Klausen J. History and physical examination to estimate the risk of ectopic pregnancy: validation of a clinical prediction model. *Ann Emerg Med* 1999;34:589-94.
8   Wong T, Lau C, Yeung A, Lo L, Tai C. Efficacy of transabdominal ultrasound examination in the diagnosis of early pregnancy complications in an emergency department. *BMJ* 1998;15:155.
9   Mol B, Lijmer J, Ankum W, Van der Veen F, Bossuyt P. The accuracy of single serum progesterone measurement in the diagnosis of ectopic pregnancy: a meta-analysis. *Hum Reprod* 1998;13:3220.

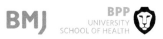

Appendicitis

Sian R R Lewis, locum general practitioner[1],
Peter J Mahony, general practitioner[2],
John Simpson, associate professor in gastrointestinal surgery[3]

[1]Nottingham, UK

[2]Belvoir Health Group, The Surgery, Nottingham, UK

[3]Department of General Surgery, University Hospital/Queens Medical Centre, Nottingham NG7 2UH, UK

Correspondence to: J Simpson j.simpson@nottingham.ac.uk

Cite this as: BMJ 2011;343:d5976

DOI: 10.1136/bmj.d5976

www.bmj.com/content/343/bmj.d5976

Acute appendicitis is the most common abdominal condition requiring emergency surgery. It results from inflammation of the vermiform appendix, which is a tubular structure attached to the base of the caecum.

Why is appendicitis missed?

The classical presentation of appendicitis appears in only approximately 50% of patients.[4] Appendicitis can affect all age groups, and presentation may be influenced by the patient's age and the anatomical position of the appendix. An accurate history may not be possible from the very young or from older people presenting with confusion.

Pregnancy seems to protect against appendicitis,[5] but it is the most common non-obstetric emergency requiring surgery in pregnancy. Presentations in pregnant women may be atypical (due to anatomical displacement of the appendix by the gravid uterus) or mistaken for the onset of labour; tenderness may be located anywhere on the right side of the abdomen or may be minimal if the inflamed appendix is displaced posterolaterally.

The diagnostic accuracy of general practitioners in relation to appendicitis is high (92% of paediatric cases correctly diagnosed) and the non-specificity of symptoms and signs is the predominant reason for a delay in diagnosis.[6]

Why does this matter?

Appendicitis is a progressive inflammatory process, and the incidence of perforated cases rises with the duration of symptoms. Therefore, prompt diagnosis and treatment are essential for reducing the increased risk associated with advanced inflammation. After the first 36 hours following the onset of symptoms the average rate of perforation is between 16% and 36%, and the risk of perforation is 5% for every subsequent 12 hour period.[7] Perforation rates are higher in elderly people and young children,[8] possibly because of a delay in diagnosis.[9] However, actual perforation rates are difficult to calculate accurately due to the frequency of undiagnosed cases of resolving appendicitis.[10]

How is appendicitis diagnosed?

Clinical features

Diagnosis of acute appendicitis relies on a thorough history and examination, and the presence or absence of any particular individual symptom or sign cannot be relied upon to diagnose or exclude appendicitis.

In the assessment of a patient with suspected appendicitis, studies have demonstrated that pain migration (positive likelihood ratio 2.06) and evidence of peritoneal irritation

---

KEY POINTS

- Appendicitis is a predominantly clinical diagnosis, and no single individual symptom or sign can be relied upon to diagnose or exclude it
- A history of fever or pain migration and evidence of peritoneal irritation have been found to be the most useful clinical features in making the diagnosis
- A raised CRP and white cell count can support the diagnosis
- The classical presentation can be influenced by the age of the patient and anatomical position of the appendix

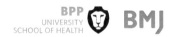

(localised direct or indirect tenderness (1.29-2.47), rigidity (2.96), guarding (2.48), rebound (1.99), and percussion tenderness (2.86) are the most useful clinical findings associated with a positive diagnosis.[11]

Abdominal pain is the primary presenting complaint of patients with acute appendicitis. However, the sequence of vague abdominal pain followed by vomiting with migration of the pain to the right iliac fossa first described by Murphy may be present only in around 50% of patients.[4] Typically, the patient describes a periumbilical or epigastric pain that intensifies during the first 24 hours, becoming constant and sharp, and migrates to the right iliac fossa. Loss of appetite is often a predominant feature, and constipation and nausea are frequently present. Profuse vomiting is rarely a major feature in simple appendicitis. The patient can be flushed, with a dry tongue and associated fetor oris. The presence of pyrexia (up to 38°C) with tachycardia is common. Abdominal examination reveals localised tenderness and muscular rigidity after localisation of the pain to the right iliac fossa. The site of maximal tenderness is often said to be over McBurney's point, which lies two thirds of the way along a line drawn from the umbilicus to the anterior superior iliac spine. Rebound tenderness is present but the test should be used with caution as it can be distressing for the patient. Movement frequently exacerbates the pain, and asking patients to cough will often localise the pain to the right iliac fossa. Demonstration of Rovsing's sign (palpation of the left iliac fossa causes pain in the right iliac fossa due to peritoneal irritation) may also aid in the diagnosis of appendicitis. In atypical cases, clinical assessment of the right groin and hip is important, particularly in paediatric patients, to rule out pathology in this region.

Scoring systems

Scoring systems have been developed to aid the diagnosis of appendicitis. They aim to estimate the probability of the condition in an individual patient compared with a large number of similar patients from which the system was developed. The best known of the several systems developed is the Alvarado score,[12] although more recently the appendicitis inflammatory response (AIR) score correctly classified a higher proportion of patients into low probability and high probability groups. The scores use history and examination findings along with inflammatory markers to achieve a summed numerical score. In a study of 545 patients with suspected appendicitis the receiver operating characteristic area for the AIR score was 0.93 compared to 0.88 for the Alvarado score (P=0.0007).[13]

Anatomical considerations in the presentation of acute appendicitis

- Retrocaecal/retrocolic (20%)[14]—Right loin pain is often present, with tenderness on examination. Muscular rigidity and tenderness to deep palpation are often absent because of protection from the overlying caecum. The psoas muscle may be irritated in this position, leading to hip flexion and exacerbation of the pain on hip extension (psoas stretch sign)

- Subcaecal and pelvic (51%)[14]—Suprapubic pain and urinary frequency may predominate. Diarrhoea and tenesmus may be present as a result of irritation of the rectum. Abdominal tenderness may be lacking, but rectal or vaginal tenderness may be present on the right. Microscopic haematuria and leukocytes may be present on urinalysis

- Pre-ileal and post-ileal (25%)[14]—Diarrhoea may result from irritation of the distal ileum. A presumptive diagnosis of gastroenteritis may delay a diagnosis of appendicitis[8]

Investigations

There is no specific laboratory test for appendicitis although simple blood tests may support the diagnosis as the majority of patients with appendicitis will have a neutrophil predominant leukocytosis. Combining C-reactive protein and white cell count can provide a likelihood ratio for appendicitis of up to 23.32 depending on values taken.[11] In contrast, when all inflammatory markers are normal, appendicitis is unlikely.[11]

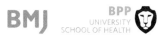

To assess for obstetric related conditions, pregnancy testing is mandatory in women of child bearing age.

Urinalysis may be abnormal in almost half of patients with acute appendicitis because of inflammation adjacent to the right sided urinary tract and bladder.[15]

Appendicitis is predominantly a clinical diagnosis that can be supported by simple blood tests—specialist tests aren't usually required. However, the most frequently used radiological investigations are ultrasonography (sensitivity and specificity of 86% and 81%) and computed tomography (94% and 95%),[16] although the latter should be used with caution to minimise radiation exposure.

How is appendicitis managed?

Appropriate resuscitation followed by expedient appendicectomy either by the open or laparoscopic approach is the treatment of choice. All patients should receive broad spectrum perioperative antibiotics as this decreases the incidence of postoperative wound infections and abscess formation.[17]

CASE SCENARIO

A 50 year old man presented with a 24 hour history of generalised abdominal pain that had become localised in the right loin. He had no urinary symptoms but was feverish (37.8°C). His urine was positive for blood and protein, and a provisional diagnosis of renal colic was made. He was referred to hospital, where computed tomography of the kidneys, ureters, and bladder did not demonstrate any evidence of urinary calculi but did confirm the presence of an inflamed retrocaecal appendix. He underwent an open appendicectomy and made an uneventful recovery.

HOW COMMON IS APPENDICITIS?

- Appendicitis is the most common abdominal emergency and accounts for more than 40000 hospital admissions in England every year (approximately 1 per 1500 population)[1]

- Appendicitis is most common between the ages of 10 and 20 years, but no age group is exempt

- There is a male to female ratio of 1.4:1; overall lifetime risk is 8.6% for males and 6.7% for females in the United States[2]

- Since the 1940s the incidence of hospital admission for acute appendicitis has been falling, but the reason for this decline is not clear[3]

Contributors: SRRL and JS wrote the first draft. PJM made important revisions. JS is guarantor.

Competing interests: All authors have completed the ICMJE uniform disclosure form at www.icmje. org/coi_disclosure.pdf (available on request from the corresponding author) and declare: no support from any organisation for the submitted work; no financial relationships with any organisations that might have an interest in the submitted work in the previous three years, no other relationships or activities that could appear to have influenced the submitted work. JS declares that MA Healthcare paid travel expenses and accommodation fees for speaking at an educational event on the subject of acute appendicitis in September 2010.

Provenance and peer review: Commissioned; externally peer reviewed.

Patient consent not required (patient anonymised, dead, or hypothetical).

1 Hospital Episode Statistics. Primary diagnosis: summary. www.hesonline.nhs.uk/Ease/servlet/ContentServer?siteID=1937&categoryID=202.
2 Addiss DG, Shaffer N, Fowler BS, Tauxe RV. The epidemiology of appendicitis and appendectomy in the United States. Am J Epidemiol 1990;132:910-25.
3 Kang JY, Hoare J, Majeed A, Williamson RC, Maxwell JD. Decline in admission rates for acute appendicitis in England. Br J Surg 2003;90:1586-92.
4 Murphy JB. Two thousand operations for appendicitis, with deductions from his personal experience. Am J Med Sci 1904;128:187-211.
5 Andersson RE, Lambe M. Incidence of appendicitis during pregnancy. Int J Epidemiol 2001;30:1281-5.
6 Wilson D, Sinclair S, McCallion WA, Potts SR. Acute appendicitis in young children in the Belfast urban area: 1985-1992. Ulster Med J 1994;63:3-7.

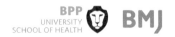

7   Bickell NA, Aufses AH Jr, Rojas M, Bodian C. How time affects the risk of rupture in appendicitis. *J Am Coll Surg* 2006;202:401-6.

8   Cappendijk VC, Hazebroek FW. The impact of diagnostic delay on the course of acute appendicitis. *Arch Dis Child* 2000;83:64-6.

9   Hale DA, Molloy M, Pearl RH, Schutt DC, Jaques DP. Appendectomy: a contemporary appraisal. *Ann Surg* 1997;225:252-61.

10 Andersson RE. The natural history and traditional management of appendicitis revisited: spontaneous resolution and predominance of prehospital perforations imply that a correct diagnosis is more important than an early diagnosis. *World J Surg* 2007;31:86-92.

11 Andersson RE. Meta-analysis of the clinical and laboratory diagnosis of appendicitis. *Br J Surg* 2004;91:28-37.

12 Alvarado A. A practical score for the early diagnosis of acute appendicitis. *Ann Emerg Med* 1986;15:557-64.

13 Andersson M, Andersson RE.The appendicitis inflammatory response score: a tool for the diagnosis of acute appendicitis that outperforms the Alvarado score. *World J Surg* 2008;32:1843-9.

14 Ahmed I, Asgeirsson KS, Beckingham IJ, Lobo DN. The position of the vermiform appendix at laparoscopy. *Surg Radiol Anat* 2007;29:165-8.

15 Puskar D, Bedalov G, Fridrih S, Vuckovic I, Banek T, Pasini J. Urinalysis, ultrasound analysis, and renal dynamic scintigraphy in acute appendicitis. *Urology* 1995;45:108-12.

16 Terasawa T, Blackmore CC, Bent S, Kohlwes RJ. Systematic review: computed tomography and ultrasonography to detect acute appendicitis in adults and adolescents. *Ann Intern Med* 2004;141:537-46.

17 Andersen BR, Kallehave FL, Andersen HK. Antibiotics versus placebo for prevention of postoperative infection after appendicectomy. *Cochrane Database Syst Rev* 2005;3:CD001439.

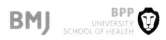

Inflammatory bowel disease

Ella Mozdiak, clinical research fellow in gastroenterology[1],
John O'Malley, general practitioner and clinical director[2],
Ramesh Arasaradnam, consultant gastroenterologist, senior lecturer[3]

[1]Gastroenterology Department, University Hospitals Coventry and Warwickshire, Coventry, UK

[2]Trafford Health Centre, Trafford, UK

[3]University of Warwick, Coventry CV2 2DX, UK

Correspondence to: R Arasaradnam r.arasaradnam@warwick.ac.uk

Cite this as: BMJ 2015;351:h4416

DOI: 10.1136/bmj.h4416

www.bmj.com/content/351/bmj.h4416

A 21 year old woman presented to her general practitioner with tiredness and abdominal discomfort for the past year. She is treated for iron deficiency anaemia (attributed to menorrhagia) and for presumed irritable bowel syndrome. After hospital admission a few months later with suspected appendicitis, tests reveal vitamin B12 deficiency and raised inflammatory markers, prompting gastroenterology referral. Colonoscopy with terminal ileal biopsy confirms a diagnosis of Crohn's disease.

What is inflammatory bowel disease?

Inflammatory bowel disease encompasses ulcerative colitis and Crohn's disease, both idiopathic chronic diseases of the gastrointestinal tract. Ulcerative colitis is characterised by diffuse inflammation affecting the mucosa of the colon only. Crohn's disease involves patchy transmural ulceration that can affect any part of the gastrointestinal tract. Around 5% of patients have features of both subtypes and are labelled inflammatory bowel disease "unclassified."[1]

Why is it missed?

Recent data on the incidence of delayed diagnosis are limited. A recent Swiss cohort study found the median diagnostic delay among patients with Crohn's disease was 9 months and was 4 months among patients with ulcerative colitis. Age <40 years and ileal disease were independently associated with a long diagnostic delay in Crohn's disease.[4]

Lower gastrointestinal symptoms are common in general practice, and symptoms typical of irritable bowel syndrome are often described in patients with inflammatory bowel disease.[5] A large UK based case-control study found that patients with inflammatory bowel disease were three times more likely to have a prior diagnosis of irritable bowel syndrome.[6] A prospective cohort study found patients with probable and possible pre-existing irritable bowel syndrome were likely to experience longer symptom duration before diagnosis of inflammatory bowel disease.[7] Onset of both diseases is often insidious, and there are no pathognomonic signs or symptoms of either. Many patients have vague, non-specific symptoms for some time, consistent with chronic low level inflammation which can mimic irritable bowel syndrome. In addition the relapsing and remitting nature of inflammatory bowel disease compounds the diagnostic difficulty.

THE BOTTOM LINE

- Inflammatory bowel disease can present with symptoms similar to irritable bowel syndrome
- Diarrhoea of >6 weeks' duration, especially with weight loss and where cancer is not suspected, warrants testing (such as full blood count, C reactive protein or erythrocyte sedimentation rate, coeliac antibodies, and thyroid function)
- NICE guidelines recommend measuring faecal calprotectin in all patients with suspected inflammatory bowel disease, as it is useful in excluding the disease
- Delayed diagnosis of inflammatory bowel disease is associated with reduced response to medical therapy and higher incidence of surgical intervention

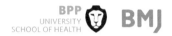

Why does this matter?

Delay in the diagnosis of inflammatory bowel disease has been suggested to reduce patient quality of life but also to reduce response to medical therapy.[8] A retrospective cohort study showed that longer diagnostic delay in Crohn's disease was associated with greater risk of bowel stenosis and of intestinal surgery for Crohn's disease.[8]

Current statistics suggest up to 50% of patients with Crohn's disease will require surgery within 10 years of diagnosis,[3] but evidence suggests a reduction in surgery over the past decade owing to treatment advances.[8] Improved remission rates and short term treatment efficacy have been observed in those treated aggressively at an early stage.[9] In addition, early biological therapy with mucosal healing may modify the course of the disease.[9]

Gastrointestinal malignancy is more common in patients with inflammatory bowel disease, and surveillance colonoscopy is recommended for patients with colitis from 10 years after the onset of symptoms. Therefore, timing of diagnosis is crucial.

How is inflammatory bowel disease diagnosed?

Clinical features

Both Crohn's disease and ulcerative colitis most commonly present in late adolescence and early adulthood, with a small second peak in the fifth decade in the case of ulcerative colitis.[10] Non-bloody diarrhoea lasting more than six weeks makes infective causes less likely and warrants further investigation.[10] Fever and anorexia are not seen in irritable bowel syndrome and nocturnal symptoms are unusual, whereas they are not uncommon in inflammatory bowel disease.[1]

Some 90% of patients with ulcerative colitis report bloody diarrhoea,[10] usually triggering prompt investigations; in addition, abdominal pain and urgency of defecation are commonly seen. Crohn's disease tends to have a more varied presentation—chronic diarrhoea is the most common symptom, but abdominal pain and weight loss are seen in 70% and 60% of patients, respectively.[11] Other patients can present more acutely with intestinal obstruction due to stricturing disease or perianal complications including abscesses and fistulas.

Between 25% and 40% of patients with inflammatory bowel disease have extraintestinal manifestations, more often affecting those with Crohn's disease. The musculoskeletal system (arthritis, ankylosing spondylitis) and skin (erythema nodosum, psoriasis, pyoderma gangrenosum) are most commonly affected and may be the presenting feature.[12]

Investigations

There is no single diagnostic test for inflammatory bowel disease: a combination of clinical, radiological, endoscopic, and histological investigations are used in secondary care. In primary care, check full blood count for anaemia or microcytosis (suggesting iron deficiency or anaemia of chronic disease) and for thrombocytosis (indicating inflammation). Check C reactive protein or erythrocyte sedimentation rate: these inflammatory markers can indicate disease activity but lack sensitivity and specificity. Exclude coeliac disease (with antibody testing), thyroid dysfunction (with serum thyroid stimulating hormone level), and infective diarrhoea (stool microscopy). As malabsorption may occur in inflammatory bowel disease, check serum B12, folate and ferritin levels, and transferrin saturation.

Faecal calprotectin is released into the colon in excess in the presence of inflammation. The National Institute for Health and Care Excellence (NICE) recommends testing for this to help distinguish inflammatory bowel disease from other non-inflammatory bowel conditions such as irritable bowel syndrome in those with lower gastrointestinal symptoms of recent onset and where cancer is not suspected[3]—that is, those without referral criteria for malignancy.[13]

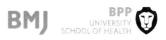

A recent systematic review has shown a cut-off of 50 µg/g of faecal calprotectin to be sensitive and specific for inflammatory bowel disease,[14] but more data are needed to determine optimal threshold values in primary care. Values >50 µg/g are not diagnostic but warrant specialist assessment within four weeks. The test's utility lies in its high negative predictive value.[14] Thus, a normal result means inflammatory bowel disease is unlikely.

Lower gastrointestinal endoscopy with histological confirmation on biopsy is considered the first line diagnostic test after referral. Plain abdominal x ray is essential if acute colonic inflammation or bowel obstruction is suspected, but is not diagnostic and not recommended for routine use.[10] [11]

How is inflammatory bowel disease managed?

Refer patients who have bloody diarrhoea, diarrhoea of >6 weeks' duration, abdominal pain with weight loss, raised faecal calprotectin, or unexplained vitamin B12 or folate deficiency in an adult <40 years old. Management is based in secondary care and made on an individual basis, dependent on disease extent, location, and behaviour with the aim to induce and maintain remission via a multidisciplinary approach. Diet and lifestyle advice (such as eating a balanced diet and staying well hydrated, exercising, and avoiding stress) is important, with smoking cessation crucial in Crohn's disease. Medical management is individualised and includes glucocorticosteroids, immunomodulators, biological therapy, and mesalazine (5-aminosalicylic acid) in ulcerative colitis. Nutritional deficiencies should be corrected. The need for surgery is declining, but currently 10% of ulcerative colitis patients will need a colectomy and up to 50% of patients with Crohn's disease will require surgical management in the first 10 years after diagnosis owing to stricturing or fistulating disease.[3]

HOW COMMON IS INFLAMMATORY BOWEL DISEASE?

- A large systematic review showed the incidence and prevalence of inflammatory bowel disease are increasing with time,[2] in particular among second generation Asian migrants in the UK

- The incidence of ulcerative colitis is about 10-20/100 000/year, with a reported prevalence of 100-200/100 000 people[3]

- The incidence of Crohn's disease is around 5-10/100 000/year, with a prevalence of 50-100/100 000 people[3]

- There is little gender difference in the prevalence of inflammatory bowel disease, but it is more common in white people

---

Contributors: EM and RA wrote the article. EM performed the literature search. JO provided a primary care perspective. All authors helped revise the manuscript. RA acts as guarantor.

Competing interests: We have read and understood the BMJ policy on declaration of interests and declare the following interests: RA received fees for educational talks from Thermo Fisher Scientific, which produces the faecal calprotectin test, outside the submitted work. JO received fees from Thermo Fisher Scientific and from Tillotts Pharma outside the submitted work.

Provenance and peer review: Commissioned; externally peer reviewed.

Patient consent: Not required (patient anonymised, dead, or hypothetical).

1 Lees C, Ho GT, Satsangi J, et al. Guidelines for the management of inflammatory bowel disease in adults. Gut2011;60:571-607.
2 Molodecky NA, Soon IS, Rabi DM, et al. Increasing incidence and prevalence of the inflammatory bowel diseases with time, based on systematic review. Gastroenterology2012;142:46-54.
3 National Institute for Health and Care Excellence. Faecal calprotectin diagnostic tests for inflammatory diseases of the bowel. (Diagnostics guidance 11.) 2013. https://www.nice.org.uk/guidance/dg11.
4 Vavricka SR, Spigaglia SM, Rogler G, et al. Systematic evaluation of risk factors for diagnostic delay in inflammatory bowel disease. Inflamm Bowel Dis2012;18:496-505.
5 Bercik P, Verdu EF, Collins SM. Is irritable bowel syndrome a low-grade inflammatory bowel disease? Gastroenterol Clin North Am2005;34:235-45.

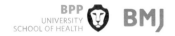

6   Card TR, Siffledeen J, Fleming KM. Are IBD patients more likely to have a prior diagnosis of irritable bowel syndrome? Report of a case-control study in the General Practice Research Database. United European Gastroenterol J2014;2:505-12.

7   Burgmann T, Clara I, Graff L, et al. The Manitoba inflammatory bowel disease cohort study: prolonged symptoms before diagnosis—how much is irritable bowel syndrome? Clin Gastroenterol Hepatol2006;4:614-20.

8   Schoepfer AM, Dehlavi MA, Fournier N, et al. Diagnostic delay in Crohn's disease is associated with a complicated disease course and increased operation rate. Am J Gastroenterol2013;108:1744-53.

9   Ricart E, García-Bosch O, Ordás I, et al. Are we giving biologics too late? The case for early versus late use. World J Gastroenterol2008;14:5523-7.

10 Dignass A, Eliakim R, Magro F, et al. Second European evidence-based consensus on the diagnosis and management of ulcerative colitis part 1: definitions and diagnosis. J Crohns Colitis2012;6:965-90.

11 Van Assche G, Dignass A, Panes J, et al. The second European evidence-based consensus on the diagnosis and management of Crohn's disease: definitions and diagnosis. J Crohns Colitis2010;4:7-27.

12 Zippi M, Corrado C, Pica R, et al. Extraintestinal manifestations in a large series of Italian inflammatory bowel disease patients. World J Gastroenterol2014;20:17463-7.

13 National Institute for Health and Care Excellence. Suspected cancer: recognition and referral. (NICE guidance 12.) 2015. www.nice.org.uk/guidance/ng12.

14 Waugh N, Cummins E, Royle P, et al. Faecal calprotectin testing for differentiating amongst inflammatory and non-inflammatory bowel diseases: systematic review and economic evaluation. Health Technol Assess2013;17:xv-xix.

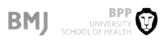

Infective endocarditis

Mark Connaughton, consultant cardiologist[1],

John G Rivett, general practitioner[2]

[1]Cardiology Department, St Mary's Hospital, Newport, Isle of Wight PO30 5TG, UK

[2]Martins Oak Surgery, Battle TN33 0EA UK

Correspondence to: M Connaughton mark. connaughton@iow.nhs.uk

Cite this as: BMJ 2010;341:c6596

DOI: 10.1136/bmj.c6596

www.bmj.com/ content/341/bmj.c6596

Infective endocarditis is caused by microbial infection of the endocardial surface or of prosthetic material in the heart. More than 80% of cases are caused by *Staphylococcus aureus* or by species of *Streptococcus* or *Enterococcus*. The total incidence of infective endocarditis has remained relatively constant, but the epidemiology has changed markedly in recent years. Proportionately more cases are now seen in association with prosthetic valves and as a result of hospital acquired infections.[1]

Why is infective endocarditis missed?

Infective endocarditis is a rare disease with varied presentations. Symptoms such as loss of appetite, weight loss, arthralgia, and night sweats overlap with much more common conditions, including occult malignancy. Fever is almost invariable,[2] but many patients may initially experience only a general malaise. Given the diagnostic difficulty, some 25% of patients take longer than one month to be admitted to hospital after their first clinical signs become evident.[2]

Why does this matter?

Data from the pre-antibiotic era suggest that infective endocarditis is almost always fatal if untreated.[3] Delayed diagnosis in some groups is associated with a substantial increase in mortality.[4] Even with timely recognition and treatment, the outcome may sometimes be poor. Observational studies report one year mortality of 20-25% and 10 year mortality of 50%, outcomes worse than for many malignancies.[5]

How is it diagnosed?

Infective endocarditis should remain part of the differential diagnosis of a persistent febrile or inflammatory illness. Ironically, once infective endocarditis is suspected, confirmation of the diagnosis may be straightforward. This will usually involve referral to secondary care, where modified Duke criteria (box 1) may be applied as the diagnostic standard. These use a synthesis of clinical, microbiological, and echocardiographic findings.[6] The negative predictive value of these criteria has been estimated as more than 92%.[7] So called "culture negative" endocarditis, which occurs in 20-30% of cases, remains a difficult challenge and may be underdiagnosed by Duke criteria.[8]

The NHS Map of Medicine suggests an algorithm for early diagnosis (http://eng. mapofmedicine.com/evidence/map/infective_endocarditis3.html) but anticipates this as taking place exclusively in secondary care.

Clinical features

Pre-existing risk factors for infective endocarditis (box 2) should arouse suspicion, but previously well individuals can also become infected. In one series of endocarditis *S aureus*, only 55% of patients had a pre-existing valve lesion and 68% of patients did not show a

---

KEY POINTS

- Infective endocarditis is rare but is fatal in about a fifth of cases
- Infective endocarditis should be part of the differential diagnosis of a persistent febrile or inflammatory illness, particularly if there are pre-existing cardiac lesions
- Diagnosis usually requires consistent clinical findings, positive blood cultures, or other proof of infection, and positive echocardiographic findings
- Treatment is prolonged and may require cardiac surgery in addition to an extended course of antibiotics

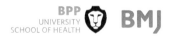

BOX 1 DUKE CRITERIA FOR DIAGNOSIS OF ENDOCARDITIS*

Requirements for diagnosis of "definite" infective endocarditis†

Pathological criteria

- Histological diagnosis from tissue, or culture of tissue or intracardiac abscess

Clinical criteria

- Two major criteria or
- One major criterion and three minor criteria or
- Five minor criteria

Requirements for diagnosis of "possible" infective endocarditis

Clinical criteria

- One major criterion and one minor criterion or
- Three minor criteria

Rejection of infective endocarditis if one of the following conditions is met

- Firm, alternative diagnosis explaining the evidence suggesting infective endocarditis
- Resolution of clinical findings of infective endocarditis with antibiotic course lasting four days or less
- No pathological evidence of infective endocarditis at surgery or autopsy with antibiotic course lasting four days or less
- The condition does not meet criteria for "definite" or "possible" infective endocarditis

Major blood culture criteria

- Two positive blood cultures for typical infective endocarditis organisms
- Persistently positive cultures for such organisms taken >12 hours apart
- Three or more positive cultures taken at least one hour apart

Major echocardiographic criteria

- Echocardiogram indicating infective endocarditis with no alternative explanation
- Myocardial abscess
- New partial dehiscence of prosthetic valve
- New valvular regurgitation

Minor criteria

- Predisposing cardiac condition
- Intravenous drug use
- Fever (≥38°C)
- Raised C reactive protein or erythrocyte sedimentation rate
- Vascular lesions including major arterial emboli, septic pulmonary infarcts, mycotic aneurysm, intracranial haemorrhage, conjunctival haemorrhages, and Janeway lesions
- Immunological phenomena, including glomerulonephritis, Roth spots, Osler's nodes, and positive rheumatoid factor
- Positive cultures not meeting a major criterion or serological evidence of active infection with an organism consistent with infective endocarditis
- Echocardiographic results consistent with infective endocarditis but not meeting a major criterion

*Adapted from the American Heart Association[6]

†Either the pathological or the clinical criteria need to be met

---

portal of entry.[8] A fever >38°C at some point is almost invariable,[2] so the absence of any fever should lead to consideration of an alternative diagnosis. Diagnostic "red flags" include a new regurgitant murmur, which is found in almost half of patients[2]; a regurgitant murmur

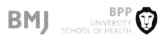

HOW COMMON IS INFECTIVE ENDOCARDITIS?

- The annual incidence is 3-10 cases per 100000

- A general practitioner is unlikely to see more than one case every 8-10 years

---

BOX 2 RISK FACTORS (AND PREVALENCE) FOUND IN PATIENTS IN EUROPE WHO WERE SUBSEQUENTLY DIAGNOSED WITH "DEFINITE" ENDOCARDITIS ACCORDING TO DUKE CRITERIA[2]

- Predisposing native valve condition (31%)

- Invasive procedure within previous 60 days (25%)

- Prosthetic valve (20%)

- Presence of pacemaker (12%)

- Congenital heart disease (10%)

- Current intravenous drug use (9%)

- Previous endocarditis (7%)

---

across a prosthetic valve; and any systemic embolus or sepsis of unknown origin.[9] In primary care, the combination of the failure of a febrile illness to resolve, together with a murmur, may be "as good as it gets" in terms of early clinical indicators. Painless Janeway lesions on the palms or soles and immunological findings such as Roth spots and Osler nodes are now rare, being found in no more than 5% of cases of infective endocarditis,[2] but they are useful if they are present and recognised.

Investigations

A definitive diagnosis of infective endocarditis will almost certainly require referral to secondary care. Initial testing in primary care may prompt earlier referral or, conversely, provide reassurance that an inflammatory condition seems to be settling. Although markers of inflammation such as erythrocyte sedimentation rate and C reactive protein are raised in over 60% of patients with infective endocarditis,[2] these tests alone are too non-discriminatory to make or exclude the diagnosis.[10] However, raised concentrations (considered to be minor Duke criteria) may aid a decision to refer. A positive rheumatoid factor is potentially useful as a minor criterion. Positive blood cultures for S aureus, Streptococcus, or Enterococcus species suggest an important infection in any context and should be referred for hospital assessment.

Positive blood cultures or other serology and cardiac imaging in secondary care are the mainstays of definitive diagnosis. Transthoracic echocardiography is readily available, but transoesophageal studies are the current best imaging modality, particularly if prosthetic material is present. Specificity for detecting vegetations, abscesses, or other evidence of infective endocarditis can approach 100%.[11] Serial studies should be performed if the initial diagnosis remains in doubt.

How is it managed?

Hospital care is mandatory for at least the initial treatment of infective endocarditis in order to assess the early response to antibiotics and to monitor and treat any complications. Little controlled trial evidence exists to guide treatment, but a substantial body of clinical experience does exist.[6] [9] Rational management involves extended courses of high dose antibiotic treatment, ideally guided by microbiological sensitivity testing. In one series of over 200 patients, 38% of patients needed surgical treatment.[5] Indications for surgery include failure to control the infection, threatened or actual embolus of septic material, and development of heart failure. Some patients may be suitable for outpatient intravenous antibiotic treatment after an initial inpatient assessment and treatment period.[9] After discharge from hospital, patients need monitoring for relapse or recurrent infection. Patients remain at risk of further episodes of infective endocarditis and should be counselled to report any potentially relevant symptoms.

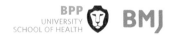

CASE SCENARIO

Four months after prostate surgery that had been complicated by a urinary infection, a 65 year old man presented with lethargy, malaise, and mild anaemia. No further specific abnormalities were found over the next two weeks. He developed night sweats, and a new systolic murmur was heard. C reactive protein was raised at 90 mg/l. Infective endocarditis was considered as a diagnosis. Blood cultures were ordered and he was referred to hospital. *Enterococcus faecalis* was grown from all culture bottles. Transthoracic echocardiography showed mitral valve vegetations, confirming the diagnosis of bacterial endocarditis.

Contributors: MC was the main author of this article and JGR contributed. MC will act as guarantor.

Competing interests: All authors have completed the Unified Competing Interest form at www.icmje. org/coi_disclosure.pdf (available on request from the corresponding author) and declare that they have no relationships with any companies that might have an interest in the submitted work in the previous 3 years; their spouses, partners, or children have no financial relationships that may be relevant to the submitted work; and the authors have no non-financial interests that may be relevant to the submitted work.

Provenance and peer review: Commissioned; externally peer reviewed.

Patient consent not required (patient anonymised, dead, or hypothetical).

1   Hill EE, Herijgers P, Herregods M-C, Peetermans WE. Evolving trends in infective endocarditis. *Clin Micobiol Infect* 2006;12:5-12.
2   Murdoch DR, Corey GR, Hoen B, Miró JM, Fowler VG Jr, Bayer AS, et al. Clinical presentation, etiology, and outcome of infective endocarditis in the 21st century: the International Collaboration on Endocarditis—Prospective Cohort Study. *Arch Intern Med* 2009;169:463-73.
3   Verhagen DWM, Vedder AC, Speelman P, van der Meer JTM. Antimicrobial treatment of infective endocarditis caused by viridans streptococci highly susceptible to penicillin: historic overview and future considerations. *J Antimicrob Chemother* 2006;57:819-24.
4   San Martin J, Sarriá C, de las Cuevas C, Duarte J, Gamallo C. Relevance of clinical presentation and period of diagnosis in prosthetic valve endocarditis. *J Heart Valve Dis* 2010;19:131-8.
5   Netzer ROM, Altwegg SC, Zollinger E, Tauber M, Carrel T, Seiler C. Infective endocarditis: determinants of long term outcome. *Heart* 2002;88:61-6.
6   American Heart Association. Scientific statement. Infective endocarditis. Diagnosis, antimicrobial therapy and management of complications. *Circulation* 2005;111:e394-434.
7   Dodds GA, Sexton DJ, Durack DT, Bashore TM, Corey GR, Kisslo J. Negative predictive value of the Duke criteria for infective endocarditis. *Am J Cardiol* 1996;77:403-7.
8   Hill EE, Vanderschueren, S, Verhaegen J, Herijgers P, Claus P, Herregods M-C, et al. Risk factors for infective endocarditis and outcome of patients with Staphylococcus aureus bacteremia. *Mayo Clinic Proc* 2007;82:1165-9.
9   Task Force on the Prevention, Diagnosis, and Treatment of Infective Endocarditis of the European Society of Cardiology (ESC). Guidelines on the prevention, diagnosis, and treatment of infective endocarditis (new version 2009). *Eur Heart J* 2009;30:2369-413.
10 Gouriet F, Botelho-Nevers E, Coulibaly, B, Raoult D, Casalta JP. Evaluation of Sedimentation rate, rheumatoid factor, C-reactive protein, and tumor necrosis factor for the diagnosis of infective endocarditis. *Clin Vaccine Immunol* 2006;13:301.
11 Rozich JD, Edwards WD, Hanna RD. Mechanical prosthetic valve-associated strands: pathologic correlates to transesophageal echocardiography. *J Am Soc Echocardiogr* 2003;16:97-100.

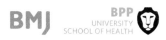

Addison's disease

Bijay Vaidya, consultant endocrinologist[1],
honorary senior clinical lecturer[2],
Ali J Chakera, specialist registrar[1],
Catherine Dick, general practitioner[3]

[1]Department of Endocrinology, Royal Devon and Exeter Hospital, Exeter EX2 5DW

[2]Peninsula Medical School, Exeter

[3]Devon Primary Care Trust, Topsham Surgery, Exeter EX3 0EN

Correspondence to: B Vaidya, bijay.vaidya@pms.ac.uk

Cite this as: BMJ 2009;339:b2385

DOI: 10.1136/bmj.b2385

www.bmj.com/content/339/bmj.b2385

What is Addison's disease?

Addison's disease (also known as primary adrenal insufficiency) is a chronic disorder of the adrenal cortex resulting in inadequate secretion of glucocorticoid and mineralocorticoid. The commonest cause of Addison's disease in developed countries is autoimmune disorder and in developing countries is tuberculosis.[1]

Why is it missed?

The onset of Addison's disease is often insidious. Its usual symptoms (such as fatigue, lethargy, weakness, and low mood) are non-specific, are highly prevalent in the general population, and overlap with many other common conditions.

Why does this matter?

A patient with untreated Addison's disease becomes progressively unwell with a markedly reduced quality of life.[5] If Addison's disease is not suspected, such a patient is often misdiagnosed as having other conditions such as depression, chronic fatigue syndrome, anorexia nervosa, or gastrointestinal disorders, leading to unnecessary investigations and inappropriate treatments. Moreover, the patient is at risk of developing serious acute adrenal crisis during an intercurrent illness or stress. Acute adrenal crisis, if not recognised and treated urgently, could be fatal.[6]

How is it diagnosed?

Clinical features

A high index of suspicion is required for the diagnosis of Addison's disease. Doctors need to be alert to the possibility of Addison's disease. A cluster of common symptoms, although non-specific in themselves, may point to Addison's disease. A cohort study of 108 patients with Addison's disease found that they had all experienced fatigue, weakness, anorexia, and unintentional weight loss.[7] Other symptoms included gastrointestinal complaints such as nausea and vague abdominal pain (56%), postural dizziness (12%), and musculoskeletal pains (6%).[7] Hyperpigmentation of skin and mucous membranes is a characteristic feature of Addison's disease; however, it is absent in about 10% of cases, which may delay diagnosis.[7] [8] Postural hypotension is common in Addison's disease; however, low blood pressure without a postural drop can also occur.

KEY POINTS

- Common symptoms of Addison's disease such as fatigue, nausea, anorexia, weight loss, and depression are non-specific, and a high index of suspicion is required for the diagnosis
- Addison's disease should be considered in all patients with persistent non-specific symptoms plus hyperpigmentation, unexplained hypotension (sitting or postural), electrolyte disturbance (hyponatraemia and/or hyperkalaemia), or a history of other autoimmune disorders
- A short Synacthen (tetracosactide) test is the key investigation to diagnose or exclude Addison's disease
- If acute adrenal crisis is suspected in an undiagnosed patient, the glucocorticoid replacement must not be delayed to carry out diagnostic tests

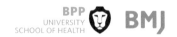

Autoimmune Addison's disease is associated with other autoimmune conditions. For example, vitiligo often coexists with Addison's disease.[7] It is important to consider Addison's disease if a patient with type 1 diabetes starts developing unexplained recurrent hypoglycaemia or the patient's insulin requirement falls as this may signal adrenal insufficiency.[9] Likewise, worsening of symptoms in a patient with autoimmune hypothyroidism after the start of thyroxine treatment should also raise the suspicion of Addison's disease as thyroxine replacement in a patient with untreated Addison's disease can precipitate an adrenal crisis.[10]

About half of patients with Addison's disease are diagnosed only after an acute adrenal crisis.[1] It is a medical emergency often precipitated by an infection or other forms of stress in an undiagnosed or inadequately treated patient with Addison's disease. In this condition, patients present acutely unwell with severe dehydration, hypotension, or circulatory shock.

Investigations

On routine blood tests, unexplained electrolyte disturbances such as hyponatraemia and hyperkalaemia may provide a clue to the diagnosis of Addison's disease. Other biochemical abnormalities, including raised urea concentration, hypoglycaemia, hypercalcaemia, and raised concentrations of serum thyroid stimulating hormone, may be present.

A clinical suspicion of Addison's disease must be confirmed biochemically by demonstrating inadequate cortisol production. Owing to the pulsatile nature and diurnal variation of cortisol secretion, random measurement of serum cortisol concentration is inadequate to assess adrenal function in most cases. A short Synacthen test is the investigation of choice to confirm or exclude Addison's disease; it is a safe test, which can be done either in primary care by a general practitioner or in secondary care via referral. In the test, 250 μg of tetracosactide (an analogue of corticotropin) is injected intramuscularly or intravenously, and blood samples for serum cortisol are taken immediately, at 30 minutes, and at 60 minutes. A rise in serum cortisol level to above 500 nmol/l 30 minutes or 60 minutes after the tetracosactide injection is considered a normal response,[1] although this threshold cortisol concentration indicating a normal response may vary according to the reference ranges of local laboratory assays. If the cortisol response to tetracosactide is inadequate, patients should be referred to secondary care for further evaluation and management. A plasma adrenocorticotrophic hormone concentration should be measured as a raised concentration will distinguish Addison's disease from secondary adrenal insufficiency. Plasma renin activity is raised in Addison's disease, and its measurement is also sometimes useful in differentiating between Addison's disease and secondary adrenal insufficiency. Once the diagnosis of Addison's disease is made, further investigations are needed to determine the underlying cause.

How is it managed?

Addison's disease requires lifelong replacement of glucocorticoid (usually hydrocortisone) and mineralocorticoid (fludrocortisone). The usual replacement dose of hydrocortisone is 15-25 mg a day, given in two or three divided doses.[1] Fludrocortisone is given in a single dose of 50-200 μg a day. During intercurrent illnesses and other forms of stress, patients should

---

CASE SCENARIO

A 34 year old woman presented with a 12 month history of increasing tiredness, anorexia, weight loss, and depression. During that period, she had tried two different antidepressant tablets without benefit. She saw her general practitioner's locum, who thought she looked tanned. Her blood pressure was 90/60 mm Hg, although it had always tended to be low. Her serum sodium concentration was 130 (normal range 135-145) mmol/l and potassium concentration was 5.7 (normal range 3.5-5.5) mmol/l. A short Synacthen (tetracosactide) test showed an inadequate serum cortisol response, which together with raised plasma adrenocorticotrophic hormone confirmed the diagnosis of Addison's disease.

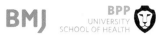

HOW COMMON IS ADDISON'S DISEASE?

- Addison's disease has a prevalence of 93-140 per million people and an annual incidence of 4.7-6.2 per million people in Western populations.[1] [2] A recent epidemiological study suggests that the incidence of Addison's disease is rising[2]

- A survey of patients with Addison's disease found that 60% had seen two or more clinicians before the diagnosis of Addison's disease was ever considered[3]

- An observational study of children with Addison's disease found that a delay in diagnosis occurred in about a third of the cases, in whom the median duration between the onset of first symptoms and the correct diagnosis was two years[4]

---

double or triple the replacement dose of hydrocortisone; this should be given parenterally if a patient cannot tolerate the drug orally (for example, during repeated vomiting). A patient with an acute adrenal crisis needs urgent hospital admission for intravenous fluid, parenteral hydrocortisone, and treatment of the precipitating cause (for example, antibiotics for infection). If acute adrenal crisis is suspected in an undiagnosed patient, the treatment must not be delayed to carry out investigations.

Contributors: BV wrote the first draft of the manuscript; all authors helped to revise the manuscript and approved the final version. BV is the guarantor.

Competing interests: None declared.

Provenance and peer review: Commissioned; externally peer reviewed.

Patient consent: Patient consent not required (patient anonymised, dead, or hypothetical).

1 Arlt W, Allolio B. Adrenal insufficiency. *Lancet* 2003;361:1881-93.
2 Lovas K, Husebye ES. High prevalence and increasing incidence of Addison's disease in western Norway. *Clin Endocrinol (Oxf)* 2002;56:787-91.
3 Ten S, New M, Maclaren N. Clinical review 130: Addison's disease 2001. *J Clin Endocrinol Metab* 2001;86:2909-22.
4 Simm PJ, McDonnell CM, Zacharin MR. Primary adrenal insufficiency in childhood and adolescence: advances in diagnosis and management. *J Paediatr Child Health* 2004;40:596-9.
5 Hilditch K. My Addison's disease. *BMJ* 2000;321:645.
6 Brosnan CM, Gowing NF. Addison's disease. *BMJ* 1996;312:1085-7.
7 Nerup J. Addison's disease—clinical studies. A report of 108 cases. *Acta Endocrinol (Copenh)* 1974;76:127-41.
8 Kendereski A, Micic D, Sumarac M, Zoric S, Macut D, Colic M, et al. White Addison's disease: what is the possible cause? *J Endocrinol Invest* 1999;22:395-400.
9 Likhari T, Magzoub S, Griffiths MJ, Buch HN, Gama R. Screening for Addison's disease in patients with type 1 diabetes mellitus and recurrent hypoglycaemia. *Postgrad Med J* 2007;83:420-1.
10 Murray JS, Jayarajasingh R, Perros P. Deterioration of symptoms after start of thyroid hormone replacement. *BMJ* 2001;323:332-3.

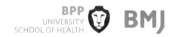

Cushing's syndrome

Julia Kate Prague, specialty registrar[1],
Stephanie May, general practitioner[2],
Benjamin Cameron Whitelaw, consultant physician[1]

[1]Endocrinology, King's College Hospital, London SE5 9RS, UK

[2]Stockwell Group Practice, London SW9, UK

Correspondence to: B C Whitelaw benjamin.whitelaw@nhs.net

Cite this as: BMJ 2013;346:f945

DOI: 10.1136/bmj.f945

www.bmj.com/content/346/bmj.f945

A 45 year old woman was being regularly reviewed in primary and secondary care because of a five year history of type 2 diabetes that had required early insulin treatment; refractory hypertension; and subsequent chronic kidney disease. She had previously described other symptoms, including weight gain, bruising, flushes, and low mood, all of which had been attributed to obesity and menopause. She was not taking any glucocorticoids. After presenting to her local emergency department with a Colles' fracture after a low impact fall, she was referred to the endocrinology department for suspected Cushing's syndrome; subsequent investigation confirmed the diagnosis.

What is Cushing's syndrome?

Cushing's syndrome describes the clinical consequences of chronic exposure to excess glucocorticoid irrespective of the underlying cause. Endogenous causes of Cushing's syndrome are rare and include a cortisol-producing adrenal tumour, which may be benign or malignant; excess secretion of adrenocorticotrophic hormone (ACTH) from a pituitary tumour (Cushing's disease); or an ectopic ACTH-producing tumour (ectopic Cushing's syndrome). More commonly, prolonged administration of supraphysiological glucocorticoid treatment (including tablets, inhalers, nasal sprays, and skin creams) can also cause the same clinical condition[1 2] (also known as exogenous or iatrogenic Cushing's).

Why is Cushing's syndrome missed?

A small single centre case series (n=33) found that the mean time to diagnosis after the first presenting symptom of Cushing's syndrome was 6.0 years,[8] during which time the diagnosis had been missed in several consultations.

The often slowly progressive, non-specific set of symptoms typical of Cushing's syndrome may not be noticed as a developing disease history in the context of many brief encounters with primary care services, or may be attributed to other common conditions, including depression and menopause.[9] Furthermore, Cushing's syndrome may mimic common conditions such as obesity, poorly controlled diabetes, and hypertension, which progress over time and often coexist in patients with metabolic syndrome or in those poorly compliant with treatment or advice.[5]

Topical glucocorticoids are commonly prescribed for eczema, asthma, and allergic rhinitis, and some formulations are available without prescription. Awareness is lacking that

---

KEY POINTS

- Consider the diagnosis of Cushing's syndrome in patients who have discriminating signs (such as early osteoporosis, myopathy, or easy bruising) or multiple features, especially if becoming progressively more severe (such as refractory diabetes and hypertension associated with end organ complications)
- Delayed diagnosis can cause life threatening illness and irreversible organ damage and may compromise the management options of any underlying tumour
- If endogenous Cushing's syndrome is suspected, refer to an endocrinologist; possible screening tests include urinary free cortisol, salivary cortisol, and an overnight dexamethasone test
- Surgical resection can cure endogenous causes of Cushing's syndrome

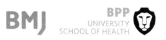

prolonged treatment with topical glucocorticoids, in all administered forms at moderate doses, can cause Cushing's syndrome.[2]

Why does this matter?

Untreated Cushing's syndrome is associated with 50% mortality at five years, predominantly from cardiovascular events (congestive cardiac failure or myocardial infarction) or infection.[10] A UK cohort study found that after treatment patients in remission had a standardised mortality ratio of 3.3, which rose to 16 for patients who had persistent disease despite treatment.[11]

Cushing's syndrome causes substantial morbidity: it can affect the musculature, causing myopathy and congestive cardiac failure; bone integrity, causing early osteoporosis; reproductive function, causing menstrual irregularity and infertility; and mood disturbance.

Delayed diagnosis can result in irreversible organ damage and in some cases can prevent the early opportunity to diagnose malignancy (for example, adrenocortical carcinoma or ACTH secretion from a small cell lung cancer).

How is Cushing's syndrome diagnosed?

Clinical features (box)
History taking
Ask about progressive symptoms of multisystem disease. A retrospective single centre case series (n=70) and analysis of other combined series (n=711) showed that the following symptoms are potentially relevant[9]: weight gain (in 97% of cases of Cushing's syndrome),

Table 1 Comparison of screening tests for endogenous causes of Cushing's syndrome

	24 hour urinary free cortisol	Late night salivary cortisol	Overnight 1 mg dexamethaasone suppression test
Rationale	Increased urinary free cortisol reflects raised serum cortisol	Assess for loss of circadian rhythm of cortisol secretion	Assess if pharmacological suppression of cortisol secretion is possible
Method	24 hour urine collection in plain urine bottle (liaise with laboratory). Collection starts after first urine of the day and finishes with first urine of the next day	Obtain sample at 2300–swab inside of cheek or swab drool until swab is saturated	Strict protocol (take 1 mg of dexamethasone at 2300 and measure serum cortisol at 0900 following morning[12])
		Specific swab is needed (liaise with laboratory)	Liaise with local phlebotomy service
		Sample can be kept in refrigerator for up to 7 days before processing	
Interpretation of result	Positive result if the value is at least as high as the upper limit of normal for the assay used[12]	Interpret using the normal reference range for the assay used[12]	0900 serum cortisol (after dexamethasone); <50 nmol/L excludes the disease
Advantages	Useful if clinical suspicion of the disease is high (specificity 91%)[13] Non-invasive	Non-invasive	Useful if clinical suspicion is low, as the test can reliably exclude the disease (sensitivity >95%)[12] [16]
		Convenient	
		Useful if clinical suspicion is low as it can confirm or exclude the disease (sensitivity 92-100%)[12] [15]	
		Specificity of 93-100%[12]	
Disadvantages	Low sensitivity (up to 15% of tests yield false negative results[14] so two measurements advised[12]) Inconvenient	Not routinely available in all laboratories	Medication (eg, anticonvulsants) may interfere with test
		Unfamiliar collection technique	False positive result in women taking oestrogen preparations
		Not appropriate for shift workers	Complicated as needs timed drug dose and blood test

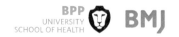

depression (62%), subjective muscle weakness (29%), headache (47%), and osteoporosis (50%). A history of diabetes (50%) and/or hypertension (74%) is probably important,[9] especially if these have been refractory to treatment and associated with end organ complications.

Assess for any possible use of exogenous glucocorticoids, especially inhalers and skin creams.

Ask to see serial photographs of the patient to assess for a change in appearance.

Examination

Look for features of the classic Cushingoid phenotype (box). The discriminant index for Cushing's syndrome is a ratio: the proportion of people in whom a clinical sign of the disease is found compared with the proportion of people in whom the disease is suspected but who, after investigation, are confirmed to have simple obesity. The higher the index, the higher the likelihood of a diagnosis of Cushing's syndrome being correct. On the basis of a study of 159 people, signs that have the best discriminatory value are easy bruising (62% of cases, discriminant index 10.3), objective muscle weakness (56%, 8.0), plethora (94%, 3.0), and purple striae (56%, 2.5).[9] Absence of these signs, however, does not exclude the diagnosis.

Investigations

Investigating for endogenous causes of Cushing's syndrome can be difficult. If clinical suspicion is high, it would be appropriate to refer to an endocrinologist for further evaluation or perform a screening test in primary care first after prior arrangement with the local laboratory or phlebotomy service. The table outlines the possible screening tests performed by specialists; these are necessary because routine blood tests—for example, random serum cortisol, liver function, cholesterol, or glucose—are not normally useful for confirming or excluding the diagnosis.[12]

If the clinical suspicion of endogenous Cushing's syndrome is high then perform a confirmatory test: either a 24 hour urine collection for urinary free cortisol (if the patient's renal function is normal) or a late night salivary cortisol if available. If, however, the clinical suspicion is low and the aim is primarily to exclude endogenous Cushing's syndrome, then late night salivary cortisol or an overnight dexamethasone suppression test would be more appropriate because of the higher sensitivities of the tests (table).

If screening tests are negative, reassure the patient but consider repeating the evaluation at six months, particularly if signs or symptoms progress.

If screening tests are positive, refer the patient to an endocrinologist for further investigation. Plasma ACTH would be measured and, if this is suppressed, imaging would focus on the adrenals (with computed tomography). If plasma ACTH is in the normal range or raised, magnetic resonance imaging of the pituitary and sometimes computed tomography of the chest and abdomen would follow, depending on the origin of the suspected tumour.

If a patient is taking exogenous glucocorticoids it is generally not possible to confirm or refute the diagnosis of Cushing's syndrome by means of biochemical tests. The clinical history and examination is therefore extremely important, and if suspicion of Cushing's syndrome is high then review the dose and duration of treatment needed.

Patients who have severe depression or who drink alcohol to excess may have pseudo-Cushing's syndrome, a condition that clinically and biochemically resembles Cushing's syndrome but resolves if the depression or alcoholism ends. The mechanisms responsible are poorly understood but are thought to involve inappropriate regulation of the hypothalamic-pituitary-adrenal axis at the level of the hypothalamus.[17] This represents a pitfall in accurately diagnosing Cushing's syndrome, and specialist advice is needed.

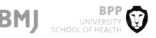

TYPICAL FEATURES OF CUSHING'S SYNDROME[9]

Features that best discriminate Cushing's syndrome from other common conditions

- *Skin*—Easy bruising, facial plethora, purple striae

- *Musculoskeletal system*—Proximal muscle weakness and/or myopathy; early osteoporosis with or without vertebral fractures or osteonecrosis of femoral or humeral head

Other features

- *Skin and hair*—Thin skin, poor wound healing, hirsutism, or scalp thinning

- *Body habitus*—Weight gain and central obesity; dorsocervical fat pad ("buffalo hump"), supraclavicular fat pads, facial fullness ("moon face")

- *Reproductive system*—Menstrual irregularity, infertility

- *Psychiatric effects*—Depression, psychosis, irritability, insomnia, fatigue

- *Metabolic effects*—Diabetes

- *Cardiovascular effects*—Congestive cardiac failure, hypertension, thrombosis (including deep vein thrombosis and myocardial infarction)

- *Immune system*—Immunosuppression causing recurrent and atypical infection, including tuberculosis

---

HOW COMMON IS CUSHING'S SYNDROME?

- An estimated 1% of the general population use exogenous steroids. Of these, 70% experience some adverse effects and about 10% have overt Cushing's syndrome[1] [3]

- Conversely, endogenous Cushing's is rare. Analysis of a national register in Denmark reported an annual incidence of two cases per million people[4]

- However, screening studies of high risk populations show a higher prevalence of endogenous Cushing's syndrome: in patients referred to secondary care for poorly controlled diabetes, prevalence was 0.6% in one prospective multicentre study[5] and 0.5% in those referred for resistant hypertension in a single centre retrospective review of 4429 consecutive referrals[6]

- Endogenous Cushing's is usually (in 70% of cases) a result of a pituitary tumour[7]

How is Cushing's syndrome managed?

Management depends on the underlying cause. Surgical resection of the pituitary, adrenal, or ACTH-producing tumour is the primary treatment of choice and is often curative.

If the disease is secondary to exogenous glucocorticoid treatment then titration of the steroid dose as soon as clinically possible is indicated. Discontinuing treatment abruptly may risk precipitating adrenal crisis because prolonged treatment may have caused suppression of the hypothalamic-pituitary-adrenal axis, so reducing the steroids to a low or maintenance dose is the safest initial intervention.

Contributors: JKP wrote the first draft, and all authors revised subsequent drafts and agreed the final version before submission. BCW is the guarantor.

Competing interests: All authors have completed the Unified Competing Interest form at www.icmje. org/coi_disclosure.pdf (available on request from the corresponding author) and declare: no support from any organisation for the submitted work; no financial relationships with any organisations that might have an interest in the submitted work in the previous three years; no other relationships or activities that could appear to have influenced the submitted work.

Provenance and peer review: Not commissioned; externally peer reviewed.

Patient consent not required (patient anonymised, dead, or hypothetical).

1 Fardet L, Petersen I, Nazareth I. Risk of cardiovascular events in people prescribed glucocorticoids with iatrogenic Cushing's syndrome: cohort study. *BMJ* 2012;345:e4928.
2 Tempark T, Phatarakijnirund V, Chatproedprai S, Watcharasindhu S, Supornsilchai V, Wananukul S. Exogenous Cushing's syndrome due to topical corticosteroid application: case report and review literature. *Endocrine* 2010;38:328-34.

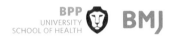

3   Fardet L, Flahault A, Kettaneh A, Tiev KP, Genereau T, Toledano C, et al. Corticosteroid-induced clinical adverse events: frequency, risk factors and patient's opinion. *Br J Dermatol* 2007;157:142-8.

4   Lindholm J, Juul S, Jorgensen JO, Astrup J, Bjerre P, Feldt-Rasmussen U, et al. Incidence and late prognosis of Cushing's syndrome: a population-based study. *J Clin Endocrinol Metab* 2001;86:117-23.

5   Terzolo M, Reimondo G, Chiodini I, Castello R, Giordano R, Ciccarelli E, et al. Screening of Cushing's syndrome in outpatients with type 2 diabetes: results of a prospective multicentric study in Italy. *J Clin Endocrinol Metab* 2012;97:3467-75.

6   Anderson GH Jr, Blakeman N, Streeten DH. The effect of age on prevalence of secondary forms of hypertension in 4429 consecutively referred patients. *J Hypertens* 1994;12:609-15.

7   Newell-Price J, Bertagna X, Grossman AB, Nieman LK. Cushing's syndrome. *Lancet* 2006;367:1605-17.

8   Psaras T, Milian M, Hattermann V, Freiman T, Gallwitz B, Honegger J. Demographic factors and the presence of comorbidities do not promote early detection of Cushing's disease and acromegaly. *Experimental and Clinical Endocrinology & Diabetes* 2011;119(1):21-5.

9   Ross EJ, Linch DC. Cushing's syndrome—killing disease: discriminatory value of signs and symptoms aiding early diagnosis. *Lancet* 1982;2:646-9.

10 Plotz CM, Knowlton AI, Ragan C. The natural history of Cushing's syndrome. *Am J Med* 1952;13:597-614.

11 Clayton RN, Raskauskiene D, Reulen RC, Jones PW. Mortality and morbidity in Cushing's disease over 50 years in Stoke-on-Trent, UK: audit and meta-analysis of literature. *J Clin Endocrinol Metab* 2011;96:632-42.

12 Nieman LK, Biller BM, Findling JW, Newell-Price J, Savage MO, Stewart PM, et al. The diagnosis of Cushing's syndrome: an Endocrine Society clinical practice guideline. *J Clin Endocrinol Metab* 2008;93:1526-40.

13 Pecori Giraldi F, Ambrogio AG, de Martin M, Fatti LM, Scacchi M, Cavagnini F. Specificity of first-line tests for the diagnosis of Cushing's syndrome: assessment in a large series. *J Clin Endocrinol Metab* 2007;92:4123-9.

14 Findling JW, Raff H. Screening and diagnosis of Cushing's syndrome. *Endocrinol Metab Clin North Am* 2005;34:385-402, ix-x.

15 Reimondo G, Allasino B, Bovio S, Paccotti P, Angeli A, Terzolo M. Evaluation of the effectiveness of midnight serum cortisol in the diagnostic procedures for Cushing's syndrome. *Eur J Endocrinol* 2005;153:803-9.

16 Wood PJ, Barth JH, Freedman DB, Perry L, Sheridan B. Evidence for the low dose dexamethasone suppression test to screen for Cushing's syndrome—recommendations for a protocol for biochemistry laboratories. *Ann Clin Biochem* 1997;34(part 3):222-9.

17 Gold PW, Goodwin FK, Chrousos GP. Clinical and biochemical manifestations of depression. Relation to the neurobiology of stress (2). *N Engl J Med* 1988;319:413-20.

Related links

bmj.com

- Chronic exertional compartment syndrome (2013;346:f33)
- Myasthenia gravis (2012;345:e8497)
- Klinefelter's syndrome (2012;345:e7558)
- Perilunate dislocation (2012;345:e7026)
- Hirschsprung's disease (2012;345:e5521)

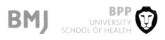

Phaeochromocytoma

Angus G Jones, specialist registrar[1],
Philip H Evans, general practitioner[2],
senior clinical research fellow[3],
Bijay Vaidya, consultant endocrinologist and honorary reader[1][3]

[1]Department of Endocrinology, Royal Devon and Exeter Hospital, Exeter EX2 5DW, UK

[2]St Leonard's Practice, Exeter

[3]Peninsula Medical School, Exeter

Correspondence to: B Vaidya bijay.vaidya@pms.ac.uk

Cite this as: BMJ 2012;344:e1042

DOI: 10.1136/bmj.e1042

www.bmj.com/content/344/bmj.e1042

A 51 year old woman presented with a few months' history of episodic anxiety associated with sweating, flushing, and palpitations. The symptoms were thought to be menopausal but they were not relieved by oestrogen hormone replacement therapy. She also had a history of hypertension that was increasingly difficult to control, despite treatment with three antihypertensive agents. Her general practitioner, concerned about a possible phaeochromocytoma, referred her to an endocrinologist. Further investigation showed markedly raised urine metanephrines and a right adrenal mass on computed tomography, consistent with a diagnosis of right adrenal phaeochromocytoma.

What is a phaeochromocytoma?

A phaeochromocytoma is a catecholamine producing tumour arising from the chromaffin cells of the adrenal medulla (85% of cases) or extra-adrenal paraganglia.[1] Although it may be malignant, symptoms usually result from the excess secretion of catecholamines.

Why is phaeochromocytoma missed?

Phaeochromocytomas are uncommon in secondary care and rare in primary care. The symptoms and signs of a phaeochromocytoma, which vary greatly, are often non-specific and similar to those of many common conditions, such as anxiety. The so called classic symptoms of a phaeochromocytoma, such as paroxysmal headache, palpitations, and sweating, are often absent. Hypertension may not be present in 10-20% of cases.[1] As a result, diagnosis is often delayed, with an average interval of three years between the initial symptoms and diagnosis, and many cases are diagnosed only at autopsy.[2][3][4]

Why does this matter?

Although we estimate from prevalence data[3] that an average full time general practitioner will have only about a 50% chance of seeing a new case of phaeochromocytoma in their career, it is important not to miss the diagnosis. Unrecognised and untreated phaeochromocytoma has high morbidity and mortality through cardiovascular complications of catecholamine excess and untreated malignancy.[1][5][6] A hypertensive crisis can be precipitated if a patient with unrecognised phaeochromocytoma is treated with β blocking medication (without α blockade, leading to unopposed α receptor mediated vasoconstriction) or undergoes surgery (which can trigger catecholamine release). Additionally, symptoms of

---

KEY POINTS

- Common symptoms of phaeochromocytoma include episodic palpitations, headaches, sweating, and psychological symptoms such as anxiety or panic
- Hypertension is present in 80-90% of cases but may be episodic
- Symptoms of phaeochromocytoma are variable and non-specific, leading to frequent long delays between onset and diagnosis
- The recommended initial investigation for a suspected phaeochromocytoma is measurement of metanephrines (a metabolite of catecholamines) in 24 hour urine collection or in plasma

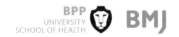

phaeochromocytoma are often debilitating and lead to poor quality of life. The condition can be treated effectively with α blocking medication followed by surgery. About 10% of phaeochromocytomas are malignant, and early diagnosis and treatment may reduce the risk of metastasis.[2] Furthermore, phaeochromocytoma can be associated with genetic disorders, such as multiple endocrine neoplasia type 2—familial phaeochromocytoma and medullary thyroid carcinoma with primary hyperparathyroidism (type 2a) or mucosal neuromas and Marfanoid habitus (type 2b). Therefore the diagnosis can also assist investigation and early identification of phaeochromocytoma and related conditions in family members.

How is phaeochromocytoma diagnosed?

Clinical

The most common clinical features of phaeochromocytoma include hypertension (80-90% of cases), palpitations (60%), headaches (50%), sweating (50%), pallor (40%), and psychological symptoms such as anxiety or panic (35%).[1][2] The combination of episodic headache, sweating, and palpitations has been reported to have high specificity (>90%) for phaeochromocytoma.[1] Other less common features include weight loss, lethargy, tremors, nausea, dyspnoea, vertigo, flushing, orthostatic hypotension, and hyperglycaemia. Patients infrequently present with a hypertensive crisis, shock, or cardiovascular emergencies such as myocardial infarction or arrhythmia. Symptoms of phaeochromocytoma are episodic in about 65% of cases, typically lasting from minutes to an hour.[2] Hypertension is sustained in 50-60% of cases but may be episodic (30%) or absent, even on repeated testing (10-20%),[1] making diagnosis potentially difficult. The National Institute for Health and Clinical Excellence (NICE) in England and Wales currently recommends that general practitioners refer for investigation if they suspect a phaeochromocytoma in a patient with hypertension, and it suggests that labile or postural hypotension, headaches, palpitations, pallor, and excess sweating are possible symptoms.[7] Worsening of symptoms after introduction of a β blocker and labile blood pressure during surgery should also raise the suspicion of phaeochromocytoma. Screening of asymptomatic patients with hypertension is not recommended owing to the high false positive rates of currently available tests.[1] On the other hand, consider investigations even in the absence of hypertension if symptoms suggest phaeochromocytoma.

About 25% cases of phaeochromocytoma are currently diagnosed in asymptomatic patients after the incidental finding of an adrenal mass on imaging performed for unrelated reasons (adrenal incidentaloma).[1] Undertake biochemical screening for phaeochromocytoma in all cases of adrenal incidentaloma.[8] Screening of asymptomatic patients with a genetic predisposition to phaeochromocytoma (such as multiple endocrine neoplasia type 2) is also indicated.

Investigations

When phaeochromocytoma is clinically suspected, investigate further by confirming the presence of excess catecholamine secretion. Measurement of catecholamines in a 24 hour urine collection has traditionally been used; however, this method has largely been replaced by measurement of metanephrines (metabolites of catecholamines) either in a 24 hour urine collection or in plasma, both of which have better diagnostic sensitivity.[9][10] Although urine collection can often be performed in primary care (unlike plasma measurement, which requires sample refrigeration or rapid processing), most general practitioners would refer for specialist advice. We recommend referral of any patient where there is high suspicion of phaeochromocytoma.

The sensitivity of metanephrine measurement to detect phaeochromocytoma is 97% for urinary levels and 99% for plasma levels compared with 86% for urinary catecholamines, among symptomatic patients, those with a previous or family history of phaeochromocytoma, or those with an incidental adrenal mass.[10] Likewise, the specificities for urinary and

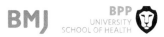

HOW COMMON IS PHAEOCHROMOCYTOMA?

- The prevalence of phaeochromocytoma in hypertensive patients attending general medical outpatient clinics is 0.1-0.6%[1]

- Autopsy studies have shown a prevalence of 0.05%, but many of these cases had not been diagnosed in life[3]

---

plasma metanephrines are 93% and 89%, respectively, compared with 88% for urinary catecholamines.[10] False positive results are common, owing to the relative infrequency of phaeochromocytoma in those tested and to the presence of other medical conditions (such as obstructive sleep apnoea) and medications (such as tricyclic antidepressants, phenoxybenzamine, clozapine, calcium channel blockers, and β blockers) that can cause elevation of metanephrines. Furthermore, severe physical and psychological stress (for example, major surgery, myocardial infarction, severe pain, panic attacks) could increase catecholamine secretion, leading to false positive results. Concentrations of metanephrines that are over four times normal levels are associated with very high probability of phaeochromocytoma; however, lower raised concentrations will require further biochemical assessment, which may include repeat testing after withdrawal of implicated medication. By contrast with the now infrequently used measurement of urine vanillyl mandelic acid, dietary restrictions are not needed when performing these investigations.

When a phaeochromocytoma has been confirmed biochemically, imaging methods such as computed tomography, magnetic resonance imaging, or meta-iodobenzylguanidine radioisotope scanning are used to locate the primary lesion and screen for metastases.

How is phaeochromocytoma managed?

A phaeochromocytoma is treated with α receptor blocking medication followed by surgery. However, because the tumour can recur even after apparently successful surgery for benign disease, lifelong follow-up is needed.[1] Genetic testing should be considered, particularly in patients under the age of 50 years, in patients with multiple or malignant phaeochromocytoma, and in those with a positive family history.[9]

Contributors: AGJ wrote the first draft of the manuscript; all authors revised the manuscript, and approved the final manuscript. BV is the guarantor.

Competing interests: All authors have completed the Unified Competing Interest form at www.icmje. org/coi_disclosure.pdf (available on request from the corresponding author) and declare: no support from any organisation for the submitted work; no financial relationships with any organisations that might have an interest in the submitted work in the previous three years; no other relationships or activities that could appear to have influenced the submitted work.

Provenance and peer review: Not commissioned, externally peer reviewed.

Patient consent: Patient consent not required (patient anonymised, dead, or hypothetical).

1   Lenders JW, Eisenhofer G, Mannelli M, Pacak K. Phaeochromocytoma. *Lancet* 2005;366:665-75.
2   Mannelli M, Ianni L, Cilotti A, Conti A. Pheochromocytoma in Italy: a multicentric retrospective study. *Eur J Endocrinol* 1999;141:619-24.
3   Goldstein RE, O'Neill JA Jr, Holcomb GW 3rd, Morgan WM 3rd, Neblett WW 3rd, Oates JA, et al. Clinical experience over 48 years with pheochromocytoma. *Ann Surg* 1999;229:755-64.
4   Lo CY, Lam KY, Wat MS, Lam KS. Adrenal pheochromocytoma remains a frequently overlooked diagnosis. *Am J Surg* 2000;179:212-5.
5   Amar L, Servais A, Gimenez-Roqueplo AP, Zinzindohoue F, Chatellier G, Plouin PF. Year of diagnosis, features at presentation, and risk of recurrence in patients with pheochromocytoma or secreting paraganglioma. *J Clin Endocrinol Metab* 2005;90:2110-6.
6   Ayala-Ramirez M, Feng L, Johnson MM, Ejaz S, Habra MA, Rich T, et al. Clinical risk factors for malignancy and overall survival in patients with pheochromocytomas and sympathetic paragangliomas: primary tumor size and primary tumor location as prognostic indicators. *J Clin Endocrinol Metab* 2011;96:717-25.
7   National Institute for Health and Clinical Excellence. NICE clinical guideline 127. Hypertension: clinical management of primary hypertension in adults (issue date: August 2011). www.nice.org.uk/nicemedia/l ive/13561/56008/56008.pdf.

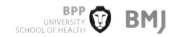

8   Zeiger MA, Thompson GB, Duh QY, Hamrahian AH, Angelos P, Elaraj D, et al. The American Association of Clinical Endocrinologists and American Association of Endocrine Surgeons medical guidelines for the management of adrenal incidentalomas. *Endocr Pract* 2009;suppl 1:1-20.

9   Pacak K, Eisenhofer G, Ahlman H, Bornstein SR, Gimenez-Roqueplo AP, Grossman AB, et al. Pheochromocytoma: recommendations for clinical practice from the First International Symposium. October 2005. *Nat Clin Pract Endocrinol Metab* 2007;3:92-102.

10 Lenders JW, Pacak K, Walther MM, Linehan WM, Mannelli M, Friberg P, et al. Biochemical diagnosis of pheochromocytoma: which test is best? *JAMA* 2002;287:1427-34.

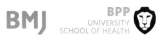

Giant cell arteritis

Nada Hassan, specialist registrar[1],
Bhaskar Dasgupta, consultant rheumatologist[1],
Kevin Barraclough, general practitioner[2]

[1]Rheumatology,
Southend University
Hospital, Westcliff-on-Sea
SS0 0RY, UK

[2]Greenbank, Painswick
GL6 6TY, UK

Correspondence
to: K Barraclough
k.barraclough@btinternet.
com

Cite this as: BMJ
2011;342:d3019

DOI: 10.1136/bmj.d3019

www.bmj.com/
content/342/bmj.d3019

Giant cell arteritis affects large and medium sized arteries, often branches of the external carotid artery but also the ciliary and retinal arteries. The symptoms are caused by local ischaemia due to endovascular damage and cytokine mediated systemic illness. There is considerable overlap with polymyalgia rheumatica: 16-21% of patients with polymyalgia rheumatica have giant cell arteritis on temporal artery biopsy, and symptoms of polymyalgia rheumatica are present in 40-60% of patients with giant cell arteritis.[1]

Why is giant cell arteritis missed?

A systematic review analysed the presenting clinical features in a mixture of studies with a total of 1435 cases of giant cell arteritis.[3] The sensitivity of individual clinical features was relatively low (table), reflecting the diverse presentation of this condition: 24% of cases had no headache at all, and only 52% had a temporal headache. Giant cell arteritis can be easily missed when systemic symptoms (such as low grade fever or weight loss), ischaemic symptoms (jaw claudication or transient visual symptoms), or polymyalgic symptoms (proximal myalgia or morning stiffness) predominate over the well known hallmark of temporal headache. The mean duration of symptoms in the 1435 patients at diagnosis was 3.5 months. A 1971 Swedish study examined 1097 consecutive autopsies with temporal artery examination carried out in each of them. Sixteen cases of undiagnosed giant cell arteritis were identified. Retrospective analysis of the case notes documented typical features of undiagnosed giant cell arteritis in 9.[4] A recent audit of 65 patients with giant cell arteritis showed that 44 had had unrecognised visual disturbance, visual loss or stroke in the mean of 35 days between onset of symptoms and diagnosis (range of 2 to 336 days).[5] Eleven of these patients presented without headache or scalp tenderness and 10 of these had visual loss.

Why does this matter?

Acute blindness occurs in up to 20% of patients with giant cell arteritis.[4] Delay in recognition may explain the high incidence of irreversible loss of vision, which is preventable with early diagnosis and treatment.[4] Jaw or tongue claudication occurs in a minority of cases but heralds a high risk of impending ischaemic complications.[6]

LEARNING POINTS

- Giant cell arteritis is a medical emergency, as irreversible loss of vision can occur in 20% of cases without prompt treatment with steroids
- "Typical" features such as headache and scalp tenderness may be absent, and this subgroup has a high risk of visual loss
- Jaw or tongue claudication occurs in a minority of cases and heralds impending ischaemic complications
- Erythrocyte sedimentation rate and C-reactive protein are normal in only 4% of cases but may be just mildly raised in a fifth of cases
- If giant cell arteritis is suspected, immediate treatment with high dose corticosteroids is indicated, and temporal biopsy should be arranged within two weeks of starting treatment

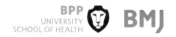

Table 1 Sensitivity of clinical features in predicting giant cell arteritis[3]

Clinical feature	% of biopsy proven cases (sensitivity)
Headache:	
Any headache	76
Temporal headache	52
Scalp tenderness	31
Jaw claudication	34
Visual symptoms:	
Any visual symptom	37
Unilateral visual loss	24
Diplopia	9
Myalgia	39
Previous diagnosis of polymyalgia rheumatica	34
Weight loss	43
Fever	42
Temporal artery:	
Pulse absent	45
Any abnormality on palpation of temporal artery (absent, prominent, beaded)	65
Erythrocyte sedimentation rate:	
"Normal"	4
>50 mm/h	83

How is giant cell arteritis diagnosed?

The typical presentation of giant cell arteritis is with temporal headache of recent onset, myalgia, or systemic malaise or fever, and the mean age of onset is 70. Erythrocyte sedimentation rate or C reactive protein is typically raised.[2] The case presented illustrates that "typical" features may be absent or subtle.

A meta-analysis looked at studies examining the value of individual clinical features in predicting positive results of temporal artery biopsy in patients with suspected giant cell arteritis.[3] No clinical features had a high negative likelihood ratio, because no clinical feature (even headache) was reliably present in all cases. Several symptoms were moderately predictive of a positive biopsy result (likelihood ratio >2):

- Jaw claudication (present in 34% of cases); claudicant pain comes on gradually during chewing, whereas temperomandibular pain or dental pain is immediate
- Diplopia (present 8% of cases)
- Any abnormality on palpation of the temporal artery—absent, beaded, tender, or enlarged (present in 65% of cases).

Other useful predictive features (likelihood ratio >1.5) were

- Temporal headache
- Scalp tenderness
- Erythrocyte sedimentation rate >100 mm/h
- Anaemia.

The limitation of these studies is that giant cell arteritis was already highly likely, as all patients in the studied population had biopsies. In practice, the condition should be suspected in anyone over the age of 50 with headache, scalp tenderness, transient visual symptoms, or unexplained facial pain. Examination may show no abnormalities, but palpation of the temporal artery is often abnormal. Only 4% of patients have a completely "normal" erythrocyte sedimentation rate (half the age of the patient, plus 5 for women[7]); 83% have a rate above 50 mm/h. Once giant cell arteritis is suspected, refer patients urgently for temporal artery biopsy, which needs to be done within two weeks of starting steroids. The true sensitivity of temporal biopsy is not known, but one model estimates a sensitivity of 87%.[8]

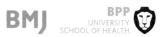

CASE SCENARIO

A previously fit and well 72 year old man presented to his general practitioner after several months of malaise and weight loss. When asked about any pain, he pointed to his left scalp as being painful. Examination was normal except that his left temporal artery was not palpable. Suspecting giant cell arteritis, the GP started 40 mg prednisolone and requested an erythrocyte sedimentation rate, which was 86 mm/h. The symptoms largely disappeared in 48 hours. She also referred the patient for a temporal artery biopsy, which showed giant cell arteritis.

HOW COMMON IS IT?

- Giant cell arteritis occurs in 2.2 per 10 000 patient years in the United Kingdom[2]

- A full time general practitioner may expect to see one new case every 1-2 years

- It is virtually unknown in people aged under 50

How is giant cell arteritis managed?

Most treatment recommendations are based on experts' opinion, as randomised trials would be unethical.[7] Once the diagnosis is suspected, treat with high dose corticosteroid immediately. Give 40 mg prednisolone daily unless the patient has ischaemic symptoms (jaw or tongue claudication, or visual symptoms). With claudication symptoms, give 60 mg prednisolone daily; if the patient has visual symptoms, admit for treatment with intravenous methylprednisolone.Once symptoms and abnormal test results resolve, the dose can be reduced in 10 mg steps each two weeks to 20 mg, then in 2.5 mg steps. Most patients have stopped taking steroids by two years.[9]

Contributors: KB conceived the idea. NH and BD wrote the first draft; KB revised it. All authors approved the article before publication. KB is guarantor.

Funding: No additional funding.

Competing interests: All authors have completed the Unified Competing Interest form at www.icmje.org/coi_disclosure.pdf and declare: no support from any organisation for the submitted work; no financial relationships with any organisations that might have an interest in the submitted work in the previous three years. KB and BD were authors of the 2010 British Society of Rheumatologists guidelines on the management of giant cell arteritis.

Provenance and peer review: Not commissioned; externally peer reviewed.

Patient consent not required (patient anonymised, dead, or hypothetical).

1   Salvarani C, Cantini F, Hunder GG. Polymyalgia rheumatica and giant-cell arteritis. *Lancet* 2008;372:234-45.
2   Smeeth L, Cook C, Hall AJ. Incidence of diagnosed polymyalgia rheumatica and temporal arteritis in the United Kingdom, 1990 to 2001. *Ann Rheum Dis* 2006;65:1093-8.
3   Smetana GW, Shmerling RH. Does this patient have temporal arteritis? *JAMA* 2002;287:92-101.
4   Ostberg G. Temporal arteritis in a large necropsy series. *Ann Rheum Dis* 1971;30:224-35.
5   Ezeonyeji AN, Borg FA, Dasgupta B. Delays in recognition and management of giant cell arteritis: results from a retrospective audit. *Clin Rheumatol* 2011;30:259-62.
6   Salvarni C, Cimino L, Macchioni P, Consonni D, Cantinni F, Bajocchi G, et al. Risk factors for visual loss in an Italian population-based cohort of patients with giant cell arteritis. *Arthritis Rheum* 2005;53:293-7.
7   Miller A, Green M, Robinson D. Simple rule for calculating normal erythrocyte sedimentation rate. *BMJ* 1983;286:266.
8   Niederkohr RD, Levin LA. A Bayesian analysis of the true sensitivity of a temporal artery biopsy. *Invest Opthalmol Vis Sci* 2007;48:675-80.
9   Dasgupta B, Borg FA, Hassan N, Alexander L, Barraclough K, Bourke B, et al. BSR and BHPR guidelines for the management of giant cell arteritis. *Rheumatology* 2010;keq039a.

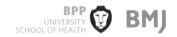

Slipped capital femoral epiphysis

N M P Clarke, consultant orthopaedic surgeon,
Tony Kendrick, associate dean for clinical research,
professor of primary medical care

Southampton University
Hospitals NHS Trust,
Southampton General
Hospital, Southampton
SO16 6YD

Correspondence to: N M P
Clarke ortho@soton.ac.uk

Cite this as: *BMJ*
2009;339:b4457

DOI: 10.1136/bmj.b4457

www.bmj.com/
content/339/bmj.b4457

Slipped capital (or upper) femoral epiphysis occurs during periods of rapid growth in adolescence, when shear forces, particularly in obese children, increase across the proximal femoral growth plate, leading to displacement of the epiphysis. The typical patient is obese. In a recent case study of 54 patients with this condition, all had body mass indexes in the overweight or obese ranges.[1] In boys, accompanying hypogonadism implicates possible endocrine causes.[2] A chronic slip is the most common presentation, with symptoms present for weeks or months as the slip progresses. An acute slip occurs after a traumatic event and prevents weight bearing, whereas in an acute on chronic slip, prodromal symptoms are followed by a sudden exacerbation of pain. The last two types of slip usually present to the emergency department rather than the general practitioner.

Why is it missed?

The indolent nature of the symptoms in a chronic slip and pain referred to the knee often mislead the doctor. Examination of the hip may be overlooked and the diagnosis missed. In a review of 106 patients, those (n=14) who had pain in the knee or distal thigh only were more likely to be misdiagnosed, have unnecessary radiographs, and have more severe slips on confirmation of the diagnosis.[5]

Why does this matter?

Chronic slippage will gradually progress in terms of severity of displacement and deformity, with increasing limb shortening and external rotation, as confirmed by a recent case series.[6] Alternatively, after prodromal symptoms, sudden severe pain may occur with minor trauma such as a fall. This indicates an acute on chronic slip, with major epiphyseal displacement and an increased risk of ischaemic injury and avascular necrosis, which can have devastating consequences. Major surgery may also be needed. Residual deformity causes femoro-acetabular impingement and premature osteoarthritis.[7]

How is it diagnosed?

Clinical features

Any child or adolescent who presents with knee pain must undergo careful examination of the hip. Loss of internal rotation of the leg in flexion, with pain at the extreme of movement, is the key physical sign.

Investigations

Anteroposterior and lateral radiographs of both hips on the same film are the primary (and usually the only) imaging needed to diagnose and evaluate the condition. Klein's line drawn parallel to the superior neck on the anteroposterior view will normally intersect the lateral

---

KEY POINTS

- Knee pain in adolescents should trigger a careful examination of the hip because it may be caused by slipped capital (or upper) femoral epiphysis
- Delayed diagnosis is associated with an increased slip and hence deformity and morbidity
- Radiography in anteroposterior and lateral planes confirms the diagnosis
- Surgical treatment of an early slip leads to an almost normal outcome

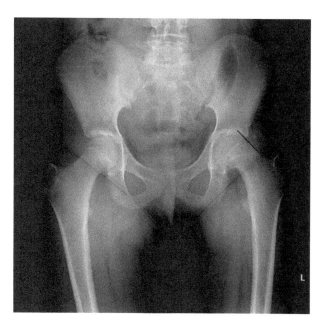

Fig 1 Anteroposterior radiograph of the hips and pelvis showing a minor left slipped capital femoral epiphysis. Klein's line drawn along the superior femoral neck does not intersect the lateral portion of the epiphysis

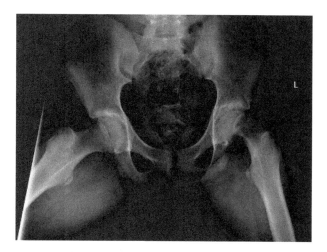

Fig 2 The same patient two weeks later, after an exacerbation of pain. The radiograph shows increased slip of the left capital femoral epiphysis, with further displacement

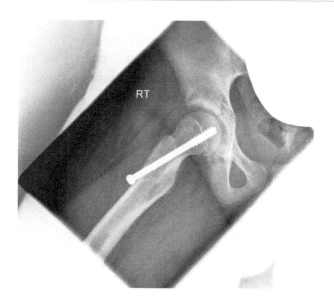

Fig 3 Screw fixation

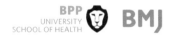

HOW COMMON IS IT?

- Incidence is 1-7 per 100 000

- It is three times more common in boys than in girls

- A bilateral slip occurs in about 20% of cases[3]

- Delayed diagnosis is common. One review of 102 patients reported a mean delay of 2.5 months and apparent initial misdiagnosis in 52% of cases[4]

CASE SCENARIO

A 13 year old boy visited the general practitioner because of a six week history of intermittent limp and pain in the left lower thigh and knee, which was exacerbated by playing sports. On examination he was overweight, but he had no abnormality in the knee. "Knee strain" was diagnosed, and he was advised to take ibuprofen and abstain from sports. Four weeks later he returned with worsening more persistent pain, now in the thigh as well as the knee. Careful examination of the hip elicited a degree of restriction of flexion and rotation, both internal and external, with 2 cm shortening of the affected leg. Radiography of the left hip showed a slipped capital femoral epiphysis.

---

portion of the femoral epiphysis but not if slipped (Trethowan's sign; fig 1).[8] Slipped capital femoral epiphysis must be excluded before investigation for other pathology.

How is it managed?

Once the diagnosis has been confirmed the usual treatment—based on expert consensus and experience—is to admit the patient urgently to hospital and place on bed rest to avoid acute displacement of a chronic slip, which can have a catastrophic affect on prognosis (fig 2).[9] Surgery is needed to stabilise a displaced capital femoral epiphysis and prevent further displacement and increasing deformity. This is achieved by single cannulated screw fixation under image intensifier control (fig 3). The more severe the deformity the more challenging the procedure, necessitating different entry points. Very severe displacement may necessitate femoral neck osteotomy or subsequent salvage procedures for persistent deformity. Remodelling can occur in younger patients.[10] Avascular necrosis and chondrolysis (chemical necrosis of articular cartilage) are the most common complications, the first usually after acute displacement (up to 35% of cases), but both may occur after surgery. Reports of the incidence of chrondrolysis after screw fixation vary, but some are as low as 1.5%.[11]

Contributors: NMPC was the main author of this article and TK contributed. NMPC is guarantor.

Funding: No special funding received.

Competing interests: None declared.

Provenance and peer review: Not commissioned; externally peer reviewed.

Patient consent not required (patient anonymised, dead, or hypothetical).

1   Bhatia NN, Pirpiris M, Otsuka NY. Body mass index in patients with slipped capital femoral epiphysis. *J Pediatr Orthop* 2006;26:197-9.

2   Aronsson DD, Loder RT, Breur GJ, Weinstein SL. Slipped capital femoral epiphysis: current concepts. *J Am Acad Orthop Surg* 2006;14:666-79.

3   Lehmann CL, Arons RR, Loder RT, Vitale MG. The epidemiology of slipped capital femoral epiphysis: an update. *J Pediatr Orthop* 2006;26:286-9.

4   Green DW, Reynolds RA, Khan SN, Tolo V. The delay in diagnosis of slipped capital femoral epiphysis: a review of 102 patients. *HSS J* 2005;1:103-6.

5   Matava MJ, Patton CM, Luhmann S, Gordon JE, Schoenecker PL. Knee pain as the initial symptom of slipped capital femoral epiphysis: an analysis of initial presentation and treatment. *J Pediatr Orthop* 1999;19:455-60.

6   Rahme D, Comley A, Foster B, Cundy P. Consequences of diagnostic delays in slipped capital femoral epiphysis. *J Pediatr Orthop B* 2006;15:93-7.

7   Carney BT, Weinstein SL, Noble J. Long term follow up of slipped capital femoral epiphysis. *J Bone Joint Surg Am* 1991;73:667-74.

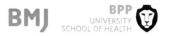

8   Klein A, Joplin RJ, Reidy JA, Hanelin J. Roentgenographic fractures of slipped capital femoral epiphysis. *Am J Roentgenol Radium Ther* 1951;66:361-74.

9   Kallio PE, Mah ET, Foster BK, Paterson DC, LeQuesne GW. Slipped capital femoral epiphysis: incidence and clinical assessment of physeal instability. *J Bone Joint Surg Br* 1995;77:752-5.

10 Jones JR, Paterson DC, Hillier TM, Foster BK, Remodelling after pinning for slipped capital femoral epiphysis. *J Bone Joint Surg Br* 1990;72:568-73.

11 Loder RT. Slipped capital femoral epiphysis. In: Staheli LT, Song KM, eds. Pediatric orthopaedic secrets. Mosby, 2007:353-8.

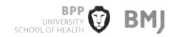

Subarachnoid haemorrhage

Graeme J Hankey, consultant neurologist and head of stroke unit[1], clinical professor[2], Mark R Nelson, chair of general practice[3], professorial fellow[4]

[1]Department of Neurology, Royal Perth Hospital, Perth, WA6001, Australia

[2]School of Medicine & Pharmacology, University of Western Australia, Perth

[3]School of Medicine, University of Tasmania, Hobart, Tasmania

[4]Menzies Research Institute, University of Tasmania, Hobart, Tasmania

Correspondence to: G J Hankey gjhankey@ cyllene.uwa.edu.au

Cite this as: *BMJ* 2009;339:b2874

DOI: 10.1136/bmj.b2874

www.bmj.com/ content/339/bmj.b2874

Spontaneous (non-traumatic) subarachnoid haemorrhage accounts for about 5% of strokes and often occurs at a fairly young age. The usual cause is a ruptured intracranial aneurysm.

Why is it missed?

Subarachnoid haemorrhage may be missed because the cardinal symptom—sudden, severe headache—is not present in a quarter of patients, and even when it is present the characteristic sudden onset might not be made known to the doctor (as patients tend to focus on severity) or the doctor may attribute the headache to a more common cause of headache with an atypically rapid onset (such as tension headache, sinusitis, cervicogenic headache, migraine) or to primary thunderclap headache, primary exertional headache, or sex headache. Among patients who present to general practice with sudden headache alone, subarachnoid haemorrhage is the cause in 1 in 10.[2][3] Subarachnoid haemorrhage may also be missed because of failure to understand the limitations of computed tomography (CT) brain scans; the sensitivity of CT brain scanning falls after the first day of symptom onset.

Why does this matter?

Failure to diagnose a subarachnoid haemorrhage is associated with rebleeding in up to 15% of patients on the first day and 40% of first day survivors over the next four weeks.[3] Up to half of patients die within three weeks after subarachnoid haemorrhage, and a third of survivors remain dependent, often with cognitive impairment.[3] Early diagnosis and referral to a neuroscience unit can improve outcome.[4][5][6][7]

How is it diagnosed?

Subarachnoid haemorrhage is diagnosed by demonstrating blood in the cerebrospinal fluid by means of a CT brain scan (figs 1 and 2) or lumbar puncture. Patients with subarachnoid haemorrhage are more likely than the rest of the population to have a history of hypertension (relative risk 2.5), smoking (2.2), or heavy alcohol consumption (2.1) and a personal or family history of subarachnoid haemorrhage, polycystic kidney disease, neurofibromatosis type 1, or heritable connective tissue disease.[8]

Clinical features

The key clinical feature suggestive of subarachnoid haemorrhage is a sudden onset of severe, diffuse headache that peaks within minutes and usually lasts one to two weeks. Although the suddenness of onset is the most characteristic feature, there are no features of the headache that distinguish reliably between subarachnoid haemorrhage and non-haemorrhagic thunderclap headache. In general practice, headache is the only symptom in about a third of patients with subarachnoid haemorrhage.[3]

KEY POINTS

- In all patients with severe headache that comes on suddenly (within minutes) and lasts for more than one hour or is associated with earlier depression of consciousness or epileptic seizures, consider the possibility of subarachnoid haemorrhage
- Refer all patients with possible subarachnoid haemorrhage to an appropriate healthcare facility for urgent plain computed tomography of the brain and subsequent appropriate management

---

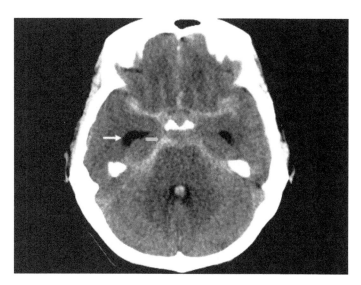

Fig 1 Plain computed tomogram of the brain showing symmetrical hyperdensity, consistent with fresh blood, in the subarachnoid space of the interhemispheric fissures and basal cisterns (blue arrow) and in the fourth ventricle, and dilatation of the temporal horns of the lateral ventricles, indicating hydrocephalus (white arrow)

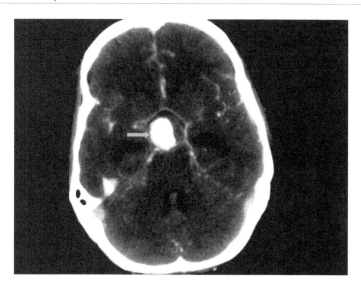

Fig 2 Computed tomography angiogram showing a large, white, contrast enhancing mass measuring 2.5 cm in diameter (blue arrow), which is central and compressing the upper brainstem anteriorly and the floor of the third ventricle inferiorly, consistent with an aneurysm of the tip of the basilar artery

Other features with or without headache include vomiting (75%), depressed consciousness (67%), focal neurological dysfunction (15%), intraocular subhyaloid haemorrhages (linear or flame shaped haemorrhages in the preretinal layer) (14%), epileptic seizures (7%), delirium (1%), radicular or precordial pain (spinal subarachnoid haemorrhage), severe hypertension, and electrocardiographic changes that can mimic those of acute myocardial infarction.[3]

An epileptic seizure at the onset of the headache is a strong indicator of aneurysmal subarachnoid haemorrhage. Vomiting is not a distinctive feature because about 43% of patients with non-haemorrhagic thunderclap headache also report vomiting at onset.[3] Preceding bouts of similar headaches are also not distinctive; they are recalled by 20% of patients with aneurysmal subarachnoid haemorrhage and 15% of patients with innocuous thunderclap headache.[3] After three to 12 hours, neck stiffness may develop in conscious patients.

Investigations
Investigations should be done after urgent referral to an appropriate medical facility. The aims of investigations are to detect subarachnoid blood and to ascertain its source.

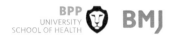

CASE SCENARIO

A 45 year old woman, well known to you as she frequently attends with migraine, has secured an appointment at the end of your Friday list. She reports her "worst migraine ever" and on specific questioning reports a sudden onset occipital headache now generalised with associated vomiting. She requests analgesia and an antiemetic so that she can "sleep it off at home" and has brought her son to drive her home.

HOW COMMON IS IT?

- The incidence of subarachnoid haemorrhage is about 7 per 100000 person years[1]

- On average a full time general practitioner with a list of 2000 patients will see one patient with the condition every seven years

- Subarachnoid haemorrhage is missed in 20-50% of patients at first presentation[2]

Detecting subarachnoid blood

Refer for an immediate plain CT brain scan all patients with suspected subarachnoid haemorrhage (including those with a rapid onset, severe headache that is maximal within minutes and lasts more than one hour without an alternative explanation).[3] The inconvenience and cost of referring the 90% of patients with innocuous sudden, severe headache for a CT brain scan is outweighed by the benefits of diagnosing and treating a ruptured aneurysm before it rebleeds in the other 10% of patients.[3]

On day 1, CT scanning detects subarachnoid haemorrhage in 93-98% of patients, depending on the quantity of subarachnoid blood, the resolution of the scanner, and the skills of the radiologist.[1] In the following days the sensitivity of CT falls dramatically as blood in the subarachnoid space is recirculated and cleared.

If the CT brain scan is normal, lumbar puncture must be performed at least six (preferably 12) hours after the onset of symptoms (unless meningitis is suspected) to allow sufficient time for haemoglobin to degrade.[8] If a CT brain scan and the cerebrospinal fluid are normal within 10 days of symptom onset, the diagnosis of subarachnoid haemorrhage can be excluded. However, beyond 10 days the sensitivity of CT brain scanning and examination of cerebrospinal fluid for diagnosing subarachnoid haemorrhage is poor, and magnetic resonance imaging of the brain is required to detect old blood in the subarachnoid space.[3][9]

How is it managed?

The management of suspected subarachnoid haemorrhage in primary care involves analgesia and ambulance transfer to an appropriate facility to establish the diagnosis and care for the patient. Supportive care includes pain relief, blood pressure control, fluid and electrolyte maintenance, and nutritional support.

Interventions targeted at preventing and treating complications include endovascular coiling or neurosurgical clipping of any ruptured aneurysm to prevent rebleeding; oral nimodipine and perhaps antiplatelet therapy and maintenance of circulating volume to prevent delayed cerebral ischaemia; thigh high stockings and compression devices to prevent venous thromboembolism; and external ventricular or lumbar drainage to treat hydrocephalus.[4][5][6][7]

Contributors: GJH reviewed the literature and wrote each of the three drafts of the article. MRN reviewed and revised the second and final drafts critically for important intellectual content. Both authors approved the final version submitted for publication.

Competing interests: None declared.

Provenance and peer review: Commissioned; externally peer reviewed.

Patient consent not required (patient anonymised, dead, or hypothetical).

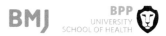

1   ACROSS Group. Epidemiology of aneurysmal subarachnoid haemorrhage in Australia and New Zealand. Incidence and case fatality from the Australasian Cooperative Research on Subarachnoid Haemorrhage Study (ACROSS). *Stroke* 2000;31:1843-50.

2   Edlow JA, Caplan LR. Avoiding pitfalls in the diagnosis of subarachnoid haemorrhage. *N Engl J Med* 2000;342:29-36.

3   Van Gijn J, Kerr RS, Rinkel GJE. Subarachnoid haemorrhage. *Lancet* 2007;369:306-18.

4   Van der Schaaf I, Algra A, Wermer M, Molyneux A, Clarke M, van Gijn J, et al. Endovascular coiling versus neurosurgical clipping for patients with aneurysmal subarachnoid haemorrhage. *Cochrane Database Syst Rev* 2005;(4):CD003085.

5   Dorhout Mees S, Rinkel GJE, Feigin VL, Algra A, van den Bergh WM, Vermeulen M, et al. Calcium antagonists for aneurysmal subarachnoid haemorrhage. *Cochrane Database Syst Rev* 2007;(3):CD000277.

6   Rinkel GJE, Feigin VL, Algra A, van Gijn J. Circulatory volume expansion therapy for aneurysmal subarachnoid haemorrhage. *Cochrane Database Syst Rev* 2004;(4):CD000483.

7   Dorhout Mees S, van den Bergh WM, Algra A, Rinkel GJE. Antiplatelet therapy for aneurysmal subarachnoid haemorrhage. *Cochrane Database Syst Rev* 2007;(4):CD006184.

8   Feigin VL, Rinkel GJE, Lawes CMM, Algra A, Bennett DA, van Gijn J, et al. Risk factors for subarachnoid haemorrhage. An updated systematic review of epidemiological studies. *Stroke* 2005;36:2773-80.

9   Van Gijn J, Rinkel GJE. How to do it: investigate the CSF in a patient with sudden headache and a normal CT brain scan. *Pract Neurol* 2005;5:362-5.

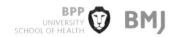

Femoral hernias

Henry Robert Whalen, clinical research fellow[1], Gillian A Kidd, general practitioner[2], Patrick J O'Dwyer, professor of surgery[1]

[1]University Department of Surgery, Western Infirmary, Glasgow G11 6NT, UK

[2]Midlock Medical Centre, General Practice, Glasgow, UK

Correspondence to: H R Whalen Henry.Whalen@gjnh.scot.nhs.uk

Cite this as: BMJ 2011;343:d7668

DOI: 10.1136/bmj.d7668

www.bmj.com/content/343/bmj.d7668

An overweight 65 year old woman visits her general practitioner with discomfort in her right groin. On examination, the suggestion of a reducible groin lump is noted. She is routinely referred to the surgical outpatient clinic with a possible diagnosis of inguinal hernia. However, two weeks later and before her surgical appointment, she again visits her general practitioner, this time with vomiting, diarrhoea, and colicky abdominal pain. She is immediately referred to the emergency department. An abdominal radiograph shows small bowel obstruction. She is admitted to the surgical ward with a diagnosis of obstructed femoral hernia and has a small bowel resection and emergency hernia repair.

What is a femoral hernia?

A femoral hernia is the protrusion of a peritoneal sac through the femoral ring into the femoral canal, posterior and inferior to the inguinal ligament. The sac may contain preperitoneal fat, omentum, small bowel, or other structures.

Why is a femoral hernia missed?

Evidence is scarce as to the reason why femoral hernias are often missed and present as emergencies. Patients may be aware of groin discomfort or a groin lump, but they may not realise its clinical importance and may be reluctant to seek medical help. Initially some patients present to primary care with vague symptoms including groin discomfort that may be attributed to other disease such as osteoarthritis. As femoral hernias are typically small, they may be easily missed on examination, particularly in obese patients. Furthermore, owing to the difficulty in clinically distinguishing groin hernias, femoral hernias may be mistaken for inguinal hernias and referred for surgical opinion on a non-urgent basis.[3]

In an emergency, patients may present with signs of bowel obstruction, which include colicky abdominal pain, vomiting, and abdominal distension. About a third of patients do not complain of symptoms directly attributable to a hernia,[4] and a groin lump is not always present. Other diagnoses, such as gastroenteritis, enlarged groin lymph node, diverticulitis, or constipation, may be made in error (fig 1).

Retrospective studies have observed that about 40% of hernias causing symptoms of acute bowel obstruction are missed owing to a lack of groin examination.[5][6] The researchers concluded that female patients and all patients with femoral hernia were less likely to have a groin examination, despite signs of bowel obstruction being noted.[5]

KEY POINTS

- Femoral hernias are more common in females and in people aged over 65 years and are associated with higher rates of complications such as strangulation
- Emergency surgery for femoral hernia is associated with a 10-fold increased risk of mortality, which is further increased by preoperative delays
- Clinical examination is unreliable in differentiating femoral from inguinal hernia
- Refer all females with groin hernia for urgent assessment and management
- Examine the groins of all patients presenting with signs of small bowel obstruction
- Ultrasound is the first line elective investigation for suspected uncomplicated groin hernia, but in acute small bowel obstruction, CT scanning is first choice

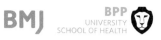

> **HOW COMMON ARE FEMORAL HERNIAS?**
>
> - About 5000 femoral hernia repairs are carried out in the United Kingdom each year
> - Femoral hernias account for a fifth of all groin hernias in females but less than 1% of groin hernias in males
> - The 40% of femoral hernias that present acutely are associated with a 10-fold increased risk of mortality[1] [2]

Why does this matter?

Although femoral hernias are less common than inguinal, they are associated with higher rates of acute complication. The cumulative probability of strangulation for femoral hernias is 22% three months after diagnosis, rising to 45% 21 months after diagnosis, whereas the probability of strangulation for an inguinal hernia is 3% and 4.5% respectively over the same time period.[7]

Several studies have shown that acute femoral hernias and their subsequent complications are associated with increased morbidity and mortality.[1] [2] [8] [9] [10] Examples of morbidity resulting from acute presentation include increased rates of bowel resection, wound infection, and cardiovascular and respiratory complications.[10] As elective femoral hernia repair has been shown to be a relatively safe procedure (even in patients aged over 80), it is generally accepted that femoral hernias should be referred urgently and repaired electively.[2] [10] [11] [12]

Missed femoral hernia at emergency presentation delays time to surgery.[5] One study has shown an increased likelihood of bowel resection if surgery is undertaken more than 12 hours after the onset of acute symptoms.[13] Preoperative delay is clearly linked with an increase in bowel resection, and this is associated with mortality rates that are about 20 times higher than those for patients having elective hernia repair (which would not require a bowel resection).[2]

How is it diagnosed?

Clinical

Classically, femoral hernias present as mildly painful, non-reducible groin lumps, located inferolateral to the pubic tubercle. In contrast, inguinal hernias are found superomedially. However, femoral hernias tend to move superiorly to a position above the inguinal ligament, where they may be mistaken for an inguinal hernia. Differentiation of groin hernias on clinical grounds is therefore unreliable, irrespective of the experience of the examining doctor.[14] In patients presenting electively, only about 1% of groin hernias in males are likely to be femoral, whereas the likelihood in females is about 20%.[1] Clinical examination alone is inaccurate in differentiating groin hernia.[14] Therefore in females, owing to the greater prevalence of femoral hernia, consider all groin hernia to be femoral until proved otherwise.

Femoral hernias may also present without a palpable lump and with only vague symptoms of abdominal or groin pain. However, symptoms may vary and there is a lack of evidence to predict the likelihood of a particular symptom indicating the presence of a femoral hernia. Patients may present later with clinical features of bowel obstruction. Undertake a detailed groin examination in all patients presenting with bowel obstruction.

Investigations

Ultrasonography, magnetic resonance imaging, and computed tomography (CT) have all been shown to be accurate in detecting and differentiating groin hernias.

Ultrasonography is widely available, non-invasive, and highly accurate in differentiating inguinal from femoral hernia—with sensitivities and specificity of 100% being reported in two studies.[15] [16] Its accuracy is, however, operator dependent.

Magnetic resonance imaging has been reported to be more accurate than ultrasonography in detecting inguinal hernia.[17] However, there is a lack of evidence for whether magnetic

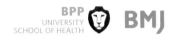

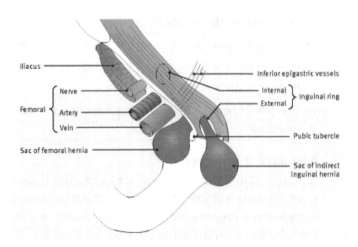

Fig 1 Inguinal hernias are usually reducible and above the inguinal ligament. Femoral hernias are often irreducible and below the inguinal ligament. Adapted with permission from Ellis H. *Clinical anatomy*. 6th ed. Blackwell Scientific, 1977

resonance imaging is better than ultrasonography in detecting and differentiating groin hernia. Therefore ultrasonography should be the first choice for electively investigating suspected groin hernia as it is more widely available, less costly, and accurate.

CT scanning has been shown to be accurate in differentiating groin hernias. One retrospective study reports the correct identification of 74 of 75 hernias (28 femoral and 47 inguinal), which were later confirmed at operation.[18] This is broadly comparable with the non-invasive modalities outlined above, but as there is a substantial radiation dose associated with CT scanning, it should not be used electively for investigating suspected groin hernia. In the acute abdomen, however, consider CT as the first choice for investigating suspected small bowel obstruction in the presence of a negative clinical examination.

How is it managed?

In males, a groin hernia suspected as being femoral on clinical examination requires urgent referral, due to the risks of acute complications outlined above. All groin hernia in females should be urgently referred for assessment.

Electively, both open and laparoscopic repair using mesh have significantly lower recurrence rates than repair using sutures only.[1] Open repair has the advantage that it can be performed under local anaesthetic. No evidence suggests superiority of either method in the acute setting.

Some research has suggested that femoral hernias may be overlooked during repair of suspected inguinal hernias.[19] So during surgical repair of all groin hernias examine the femoral canal if an obvious inguinal hernia is not observed.

Contributors: The authors jointly developed the idea for the manuscript, interpreted data from the literature, and drafted and revised the manuscript. All authors approved the final version. PJO'D is the guarantor.

Competing interests: All authors have completed the ICMJE uniform disclosure form at www.icmje. org/coi_disclosure.pdf (available on request from the corresponding author) and declare: no support from any organisation for the submitted work; no financial relationships with any organisations that might have an interest in the submitted work in the previous three years; no other relationships or activities that could appear to have influenced the submitted work.

Provenance and peer review: Commissioned; externally peer reviewed.

Patient consent not required (patient anonymised, dead, or hypothetical).

1   Dahlstrand U, Wollert S, Nordin P, Sandblom G, Gunnarsson U. Emergency femoral hernia repair. A study based on a national register. *Ann Surg* 2009;249:672-6.
2   Nilsson H, Styliandis G, Haapamaki M, Nilsson E, Nordin P. Mortality after groin hernia surgery. *Ann Surg* 2007;245:656-60.
3   McEntee GP, O'Carroll A, Mooney B, Egan TJ, Delaney PV. Timing of strangulation in adult hernias. *Br J Surg* 1989;76:725-6.

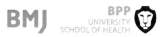

4   Hjaltson E. Incarcerated hernia. *Acta Chir Scand* 1981;147:263-7.

5   Nilsson H, Nilsson E, Angeras U, Nordin P. Mortality after groin hernia surgery: delay of treatment and cause of death. *Hernia* 2011;15:301-7.

6   Kjaergaard J, Nielsen M, Kehlet M. Mortality following emergency groin hernia surgery in Denmark. *Hernia* 2010;14:351-5.

7   Gallegos NC, Dawson J, Jarvis M, Hobsley M. Risk of strangulation in groin hernias. *Br J Surg* 1991;78:1171-3.

8   Malek S, Torella F, Edwards P. Emergency repair of groin hernia: outcome and implications for elective surgery waiting times. *Int J Clin Pract* 2004;58:207-9.

9   Andrews NJ. Presentation and outcome of strangulated external hernia in a district general hospital. *Br J Surg* 1981;68:329-32.

10   Alvarez J, Baldonedo R, Bear I, Solis J, Alvarex P, Jorge J. Incarcerated groin hernias in adults: presentation and outcome. *Hernia* 2004;8:121-6.

11   Kemler M, Oostvogel J. Femoral hernia: is a conservative policy justified? *Eur J Surg* 1997;163:187-90.

12   Glassow F. Femoral hernia: review of 2105 repairs in a 17 year period. *Am J Surg* 1985;150:353-6.

13   Tanaka N, Uchida N, Ogihara H, Sasamoto H, Kato H. Clinical study of inguinal and femoral incarcerated hernias. *Surg Today* 2010;40:1144-7.

14   Hair A, Paterson C, O'Dwyer PJ. Diagnosis of a femoral hernia in the elective setting. *J R Coll Surg Edinb* 2001;46:117-8.

15   Bradley M, Morgan D, Pentlow B, Roe A. The groin hernia—an ultrasound diagnosis. *Ann R Coll Surg Engl* 2003;85:178-80.

16   Djuric-Stefanovic A, Saranovic D, Ivanovic A, Masulovic D, Zuvela M, Bjelovic M, et al. The accuracy of ultrsonography in classification of groin hernias according to the criteria of the unified classification system. *Hernia* 2008;12:395-400.

17   Van de Berg J, de Valois J, Go P, Rosenbusch G. Detection of groin hernia with physical examination, ultrasound and MRI compared with laparoscopic findings. *Invest Radiol* 1999;34:739-43.

18   Kitami M, Takase K, Tsuboi M, Hakamatsuka T, Yamada T, Takahashi S. Differentiation of femoral and inguinal hernias on the basis of anteroposterior relationship to the inguinal ligament on multidimensional computed tomography. *J Comput Assist Tomogr* 2009;33:678-81.

19   Mikkelsen T, Bay-Nielsen M, Kehlet H. Risk of femoral hernia after inguinal herniorrhaphy. *Br J Surg* 2002;89:486-8.

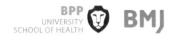

Pre-eclampsia

David Williams, consultant obstetric physician[1],
Naomi Craft, general practitioner[2]

[1]University College London Hospital, London WC1E 6AU, UK

[2]53 New Cavendish Street, London W1G 9TQ

Correspondence to: D Williams d.j.williams@ucl.ac.uk

Cite this as: BMJ 2012;345:e4437

DOI: 10.1136/bmj.e4437

www.bmj.com/content/345/bmj.e4437

A 36 year old primigravida woman attended for antenatal care at 10 weeks' gestation with a blood pressure 120/80 mm Hg and no proteinuria. At 28 weeks, she presented to her general practitioner with urinary frequency and mild dysuria. Urine analysis showed 3+ proteinuria, and her blood pressure was 144/90 mm Hg. The fundal height measured 3 cm less than expected for this gestation. A midstream urine sample was sent for culture and a review arranged for a week later. At 29 weeks, her blood pressure was 175/115 mm Hg, proteinuria was 3+, and no urinary infection had been isolated. She was urgently admitted to hospital, but on arrival no fetal heartbeat could be detected. Labour was induced and a growth restricted, stillborn infant was delivered. Maternal hypertension persisted postpartum.

What is pre-eclampsia?

Pre-eclampsia is defined by the gestational onset of hypertension and proteinuria.[1] It is, however, a multisystem disorder that can affect all maternal organs.[1] [2] Delivery of the fetus and placenta remains the only cure, but preterm delivery may adversely affect neonatal outcome, with complications resulting from prematurity and low birth weight.[3] Pre-eclampsia evolves into eclampsia when maternal seizures develop. Eclampsia is rare in well resourced countries—just 1% of all women with pre-eclampsia develop eclampsia.[4] A severe form of pre-eclampsia characterised by microangiopathic haemolytic anaemia is often termed the HELLP (Haemolysis, Elevated Liver enzymes, and Low Platelets) syndrome.[2]

How common is pre-eclampsia?

Pre-eclampsia predominantly affects women in their first pregnancy (2-8% of first pregnancies)[5] and has a variable incidence across nations, being most common in Latin America and the Caribbean.[6] In the United Kingdom, about one in 200 pregnancies is affected by severe pre-eclampsia (about 3500 cases a year).[7]

Why is pre-eclampsia missed?

Pre-eclampsia is usually asymptomatic until it is in an advanced state,[2] [8] [9] [10] and so it can evolve unchecked until the maternal condition has deteriorated to the point of severe organ failure and/or in utero death of the fetus.

In our case study, a urinary tract infection was suspected at 28 weeks, but a urinary tract infection rarely causes >1+ proteinuria. The significance of new onset proteinuria,

---

KEY POINTS

- For pregnant women with new onset hypertension (>140/90 mm Hg) and ≥1+ proteinuria, or other features of the multisystem disorder that might suggest pre-eclampsia in the second half of pregnancy, referral to their hospital maternity unit for immediate assessment is needed

- Pre-eclampsia can be life threatening to the mother (with complications such as cerebral haemorrhage resulting from uncontrolled hypertension) and to the fetus (with complications of prematurity and low birth weight)

- Pre-eclampsia is unpredictable and usually asymptomatic until the condition is advanced. It can evolve rapidly, requiring urgent delivery within hours of diagnosis, or progress slowly over weeks with conservative management

- Women who have had pre-eclampsia are at increased risk of chronic hypertension and cardiovascular disease in later life

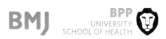

hypertension, and reduced fetal growth was not understood. This woman should have been referred to hospital at 28 weeks' gestation for further assessment of suspected pre-eclampsia and fetal wellbeing.[9] [10]

Why does it matter?
The last triennial audit of maternal deaths in the UK reported 22 deaths from pre-eclampsia, of which 20 were associated with substandard care and 14 were thought to be avoidable.[11] The most common cause of maternal death was cerebral haemorrhage secondary to uncontrolled systolic hypertension. Four maternal deaths were attributed to general practitioners' errors, including inappropriate urological referral for proteinuria, outpatient treatment of hypertension alone, and referral to a midwife for follow-up of jaundice that evolved into the HELLP syndrome.[11]

Life threatening maternal complications include uncontrolled hypertension and cerebrovascular accident; eclampsia; placental abruption; hepatic infarction and rupture; disseminated intravascular coagulation; pulmonary oedema; and renal failure.[7]

How is pre-eclampsia diagnosed?

Clinical
Guideline bodies advise a diagnosis of pre-eclampsia when blood pressure is >140/90 mm Hg in the second half of pregnancy, with ≥1+ proteinuria on reagent stick testing, which is confirmed by a protein:creatinine ratio of >30 mg/mmol.[1] [9] New onset hypertension without proteinuria but with other maternal organ dysfunction, such as thrombocytopenia or raised liver enzyme values, may also indicate pre-eclampsia.[1] Some women have an isolated rise in blood pressure without proteinuria or other evidence of multisystem disorder of pre-eclampsia, and this is known as gestational hypertension. About 20% of women with gestational hypertension will go on to develop pre-eclampsia, especially if hypertension develops before 34 weeks.[12]

In the second half of pregnancy, the following symptoms should alert the clinician to check for hypertension and proteinuria: severe headache, with or without visual aura; epigastric pain, with or without nausea and vomiting; and sudden facial, hand, and feet oedema.[8] [9] [10]

Women with pre-existing cardiovascular risk factors such as chronic hypertension, diabetes mellitus, obesity (body mass index (kg/m²) >35 at presentation), renal impairment, older mothers (>40 years old), and those who had pre-eclampsia in a previous pregnancy or who have a family history of pre-eclampsia (mother or sister) are at high risk of developing pre-eclampsia themselves.[2] [9] [10] Underlying chronic hypertension can be masked during the first half of pregnancy by gestational vasodilatation.

Investigations
For pregnant women with new onset hypertension (>140/90 mm Hg) and new onset proteinuria (≥1+ proteinuria on reagent stick testing) after 20 weeks' gestation, conduct the following investigations[1] [9] [10]:

Full blood count—To look for platelet consumption (platelets <100×10⁹/L) and haemolysis (anaemia with fragmented red cells). In pre-eclampsia the haemoglobin concentration is generally mildly raised (>120 g/L) owing to haemoconcentration

Urea and electrolytes—To look for renal dysfunction (raised serum creatinine concentration >90 μmol/L)

Liver enzymes—To look for transaminitis (alanine aminotransferase >32 IU/L; aspartate aminotransferase >30 IU/L)

Urine sample or 24 h urine collection—To quantify clinically significant proteinuria (ratio of protein to creatinine >30 mg/mmol) or 24 hour urine collection >300 mg)

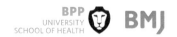

Assessment of fetus—Ultrasound assessment of fetal growth and the volume of amniotic fluid; and Doppler velocimetry of umbilical arteries.

The results of these blood and urine tests are needed within hours. As it can take several days for blood test results to be received in primary care, general practitioners should send patients to their local maternity hospital for these investigations, as well as for fetal assessment.

Pre-eclampsia can be difficult to diagnose in women with pre-existing hypertension, especially if there is pre-existing renal disease with proteinuria. Under these circumstances, pre-eclampsia can evolve in the second half of pregnancy with a surge in blood pressure or proteinuria, but more usually other elements of this multiorgan syndrome are apparent, such as thrombocytopenia, raised level of liver transaminases, and reduced fetal growth. The uric acid level is often raised in women with pre-eclampsia, but in isolation it is of poor predictive and diagnostic value and should not be tested.[9] [10]

How is pre-eclampsia managed?

Pre-eclampsia may progress unpredictably, within hours or over weeks. NICE guidelines therefore recommend immediate hospital referral for assessment of mother and fetus, with conservative management in a hospital that has facilities for emergency delivery and resuscitation of pre-term infants.[9]

Delivery of the placenta remains the only cure for pre-eclampsia. Childbirth should be considered if pre-eclampsia is identified after 37 weeks' gestation.[13] At 34-37 weeks' gestation, the decision to deliver is a clinical judgment that must weigh the risks to the mother of prolonging the pregnancy against the benefits for the preterm fetus.

Before 34 weeks, clinicians should try to prolong the pregnancy for the benefit of fetal maturity. This involves antihypertensive treatment with nifedipine slow release, labetolol, or methyldopa to keep the blood pressure between 130/80 mm Hg and 150/100 mm Hg.[9] There is little evidence to support choosing any one of these antihypertensive agents over another.[9] [10] Magnesium sulphate will reduce the risk of eclamptic seizures,[4] and monitoring the fetal condition will guide the decision for timing of delivery.[9] Antenatal administration of corticosteroids will improve fetal lung maturity in anticipation of preterm delivery.[14]

Maternal hypertension usually recovers within two to three weeks of delivery but can take up to three months.[15] Pre-eclampsia will recur in about 15% of women who had pre-eclampsia in their first pregnancy, although this risk may be as high as 25% if the pre-eclampsia led to birth before 34 weeks and as high as 50% if birth was before 28 weeks.[16] Daily low dose aspirin (75-100 mg) from before 16 weeks' gestation in future pregnancies reduces the risk of recurrent, severe pre-eclampsia.[17]

Some women will continue to have hypertension three months after childbirth. This is presumed to be the result of previously unidentified chronic hypertension or secondary causes of hypertension.[18] Even those who have made a full recovery from pre-eclampsia are nevertheless at risk of hypertension and heart disease in later life.[19] Although the optimal follow-up regimen to minimise the risk of future cardiovascular disease is currently unclear,[9] [10] pragmatic steps in primary care include encouraging optimal weight range through diet and exercise, and regular screening for hypertension, hyperlipidaemia, and diabetes.

A proportion of DW's salary is received by University College London Hospital from the Department of Health's National Institute for Health Research.

Contributors: Both authors contributed to the planning, drafting, revising, and final approval of the article. DW is the guarantor.

Competing interests: Both authors have completed the ICMJE uniform disclosure form at www.icmje. org/coi_disclosure.pdf (available on request from the corresponding author) and declare: no support from any organisation for the submitted work; no financial relationships with any organisations that might have an interest in the submitted work in the previous three years; no other relationships or activities that could appear to have influenced the submitted work.

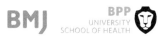

Provenance and peer review: Commissioned; externally peer reviewed.

Patient consent not required (patient anonymised, dead, or hypothetical).

1   Lowe SA, Brown MA, Dekker GA, Gatt S, McLintock CK, McMahon LP, et al. Guidelines for the management of hypertensive disorders of pregnancy 2008. *Aust N Z J Obstet Gynaecol* 2009;49:242-6.
2   Steegers EA, von Dadelszen P, Duvekot JJ, Pijenborg R. Pre-eclampsia. *Lancet* 2010;376:631-44.
3   Ray JG, Burrows RF, Burrows EA, Vermeulen MJ. MOS HIP: McMaster outcome study of hypertension in pregnancy. *Early Human Development* 2001;64:129-43.
4   Altman D, Carroli G, Duley L, Farrell B, Moodley J, Neilson J, et al. Do women with pre-eclampsia, and their babies, benefit from magnesium sulphate? The Magpie Trial: a randomized placebo-controlled trial. *Lancet* 2002;359:1877-90.
5   Duley L. The global impact of pre-eclampsia and eclampsia. *Semin Perinatol* 2009;33:130-7.
6   Khan KS, Wojdyla D, Say L, Gulmezoglu AM, van Look PF. WHO analysis of causes of maternal death: a systematic review. *Lancet* 2006;367:1066-74.
7   Tuffnell DJ, Jankowicz D, Lindow SW, Lyons G, Mason GC, Russell IF, et al. Outcomes of severe pre-eclampsia/eclampsia in Yorkshire 1999/2003. *BJOG* 2005;112:875-80.
8   Cavkaytar S, Ugurlu EN, Karaer A, Tapisiz OL, Danisman N. Are clinical symptoms more predictive than laboratory parameters for adverse maternal outcome in HELLP syndrome? *Acta Obstet Gynecol Scand* 2007;86:648-51.
9   Visintin C, Mugglestone MA, Almerie MQ, Nherera LM, James D, Walkinshaw S; Guideline Development Group. Management of hypertensive disorders during pregnancy: summary of NICE guidance. *BMJ* 2010;341:c2207.
10 Milne F, Redman C, Walker J, Baker P, Black R, Blincowe J, et al. Assessing the onset of pre-eclampsia in the hospital day unit: summary of the pre-eclampsia guideline (PRECOG II). *BMJ* 2009;339:b3129.
11 Saving mothers' lives. Reviewing maternal deaths to make motherhood safer: 2006-2008. *BJOG* 2011;118(suppl 1):1-205. (Eighth report of the confidential enquiries into maternal deaths in the United Kingdom.)
12 Saudan P, Brown MA, Buddle ML, Jones M. Does gestational hypertension become pre-eclampsia? *Br J Obstet Gynaecol* 1998;105:1177-84.
13 Koopmans CM, Bijlenga D, Groen H, Vijgen SMC, Aarnoudse JG, Bekedam DJ, et al. Induction of labour versus expectant monitoring for gestational hypertension or mild pre-eclampsia after 36 weeks' gestation (HYPITAT): a multicentre, open-label randomised controlled trial. *Lancet* 2009;374;979-88.
14 Roberts D, Dalziel S. Antenatal corticosteroids for accelerating fetal lung maturation for women at risk of preterm birth. *Cochrane Database Syst Rev* 2006;3:CD004454.
15 Ferrazzani S, de Carolis S, Pomini F, Testa AC, Mastromarino C, Caruso A. The duration of hypertension in the puerperium of preeclamptic women: relationship with renal impairment and week of delivery. *Am J Obstet Gynecol* 1994;171:506-12.
16 Hernandez-Diaz S, Toh S, Cnattingius S. Risk of pre-eclampsia in first and subsequent pregnancies: prospective cohort study. *BMJ* 2009;338:b2255.
17 Roberge S, Giguere Y, Villa P, Nicolaides K, Vainio M, Forest JC, et al. Early administration of low-dose aspirin for the prevention of severe and mild pre-eclampsia: a systematic review and meta-analysis. *Am J Perinatol* 2012;Apr 11.[Epub ahead of print.]
18 Sibai BM. Etiology and management of postpartum hypertension-preeclampsia. *Am J Obstet Gynecol* 2012;206:470-5.
19 Bellamy L, Casas J-P, Hingorani AD, Williams DJ. Pre-eclampsia and the risk of cardiovascular disease and cancer in later life: systematic review and meta-analysis. *BMJ* 2007;335:974.

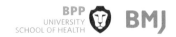

Acute Achilles tendon rupture

Dishan Singh, consultant orthopaedic surgeon

Foot and Ankle
Unit, Royal National
Orthopaedic Hospital,
Stanmore, UK

Correspondence to:
dishan.singh@rnoh.nhs.
uk

Cite this as: *BMJ*
2015;351:h4722

DOI: 10.1136/bmj.h4722

www.bmj.com/
content/351/bmj.h4722

While playing tennis, a healthy 35 year old man felt as though he had been hit on the back of the lower leg by his opponent's racquet. He couldn't keep playing but could walk. He presents the next day with mild bruising, swelling, and weakness while walking. He can walk on tip toes but Simmonds' triad (calf squeeze, altered angle of declination, and palpable gap) confirms the diagnosis of a ruptured Achilles tendon.

What is an Achilles tendon rupture?

A rupture of the Achilles tendon (fig 1) is a disruption in the conjoined tendon of the gastrocnemius and soleus muscles, usually about 2-6 cm proximal to the tendon insertion into the calcaneus.[1] Risk factors include increasing age, Achilles tendonopathy, systemic corticosteroids, previous steroid injections into or around the Achilles tendon, and use of quinolone antibiotics.[1][2]

Why is it missed?

A non-specialist may miss the diagnosis in around 20% of cases for several reasons.[5][6] The patient may rationalise the injury as a direct blow, leading the clinician to suspect local bruising rather than a rupture.[5] The clinician may regard the injury as trivial because a history on an audible snap may not be elicited, about a third of patients with complete tendon rupture do not mention pain,[7] external bruising and swelling may be mild (as the tendon usually ruptures within its paratenon sheath), a gap may not be evident in longitudinal tears (fig 2) or with swelling or bleeding, and other plantarflexors may mask the weakness from a ruptured Achilles tendon (fig 3). Thus, a patient being able to walk, stand on tiptoes, and plantarflex the ankle against resistance can lull the clinician into missing the diagnosis.[5]

Why does this matter?

Treatment delay leads to poorer outcomes,[1][8] as a discontinuous or lengthened tendon (fig 4) can cause weak plantar flexion, fatigue, limp, and inability to run, heel rise, play sports, and climb stairs.[8] More complicated surgery, with longer scars and higher risks of complications, may be required, and return to sports is not always possible.[8]

How is it diagnosed?

Clinical features

Patients with acute ruptures generally describe feeling a sudden painful blow to the heel, sometimes accompanied by an audible snap, during sports or running. They may wrongly believe that they have been kicked or hit on the back of the heel tendon by a ball or racquet. They experience residual calf ache, mild bruising, swelling, and a weakness in "pushing off" with the affected foot.

On examination, ask the patient to lie prone on an examination couch with feet dangling over the edge. Use of Simmonds' triad (angle of declination, palpation for a gap, and calf squeeze; see fig 5 and video at https://youtu.be/8PvgvUV8N8U),[9] yields a more accurate diagnosis than Thomson's calf squeeze test alone.[10][11]

Simmonds' triad:

Look (inspect for angle of declination of the foot)—The altered angle of declination (or "angle of dangle") refers to the loss of tension in a ruptured Achilles tendon, which causes the injured ankle and foot to lie in a more dorsiflexed position than the

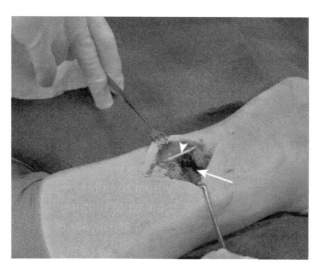

Fig 1 On opening the paratenon at surgery, the two ends of a complete transverse rupture of the Achilles tendon, with an intervening gap (arrow), are seen. The plantaris tendon is intact (arrowhead)

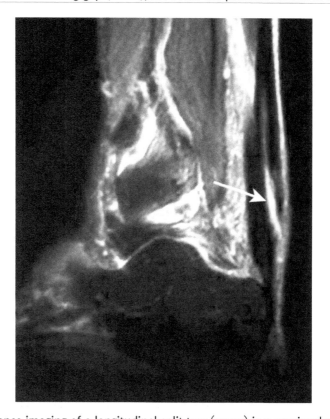

Fig 2 Magnetic resonance imaging of a longitudinal split tear (arrow) in a previously tendonopathic Achilles tendon. No gap in the tendon is evident on palpation

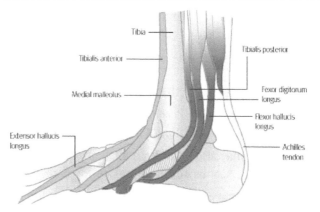

Fig 3 Other tendons (in red) such as the tibialis posterior tendon and the toe flexors can plantarflex the ankle, thus enabling a patient to walk on tiptoes even if the Achilles tendon is ruptured

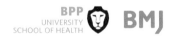

uninjured one. This test was modified by Matles,[12] who asked the patient to actively flex the knee through 90° while observing whether the foot of the injured leg falls into a more dorsiflexed position. The Matles test alone has a sensitivity of 0.88 and a positive predictive value of 0.92.[11]

Feel (palpate for a gap)—A gap can often be discerned by palpating the tendon along its entire length; the sensitivity is only 0.73 and the positive predictive value is 0.82.[11]

Move (calf squeeze)—The examiner sequentially gently squeezes the patient's calf muscles: squeezing the calf deforms the soleus muscle, causing the overlying gastrocnemius-soleus tendon to bow away from the tibia, resulting in plantar flexion of the foot if the tendon is intact.[13] If there is an acute rupture, the injured foot remains in its neutral position on squeezing the calf, with a sensitivity of 0.96 and a positive predictive value of 0.98.[11]

The Simmonds triad is preferred to Thomson's isolated calf squeeze test,[10] as a comparative study found that two of the three tests (palpation, Matles test, and calf squeeze) were positive in all ruptures, suggesting a sensitivity of 100% for this triad.[11]

Record calf squeeze findings as "plantarflexion noted" or "plantarflexion not noted" (since "calf squeeze test positive" could mean either positive plantarflexion or positive rupture).

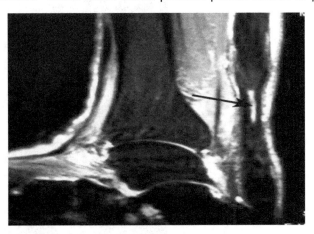

Fig 4 Magnetic resonance imaging of a missed rupture at six weeks shows that the two ends of the Achilles tendon have retracted and the gap is filled with a flimsy pseudotendon (arrow), leading to a lengthened and weakened tendon

---

WHAT YOU NEED TO KNOW

- Patients with an Achilles tendon rupture often report feeling a blow to the heel and sometimes an audible snap while playing sports or running

- Patients may still be able to walk on tiptoes and plantarflex against resistance because the other ankle plantarflexors are intact

- The Simmonds' triad of altered angle of declination (the foot of the injured leg rests in a more dorsiflexed position than the other side when the patient lies prone), palpable gap, and lack of plantarflexion on calf squeeze test will detect a rupture in nearly all cases

- Imaging is rarely necessary

HOW COMMON IS ACUTE ACHILLES TENDON RUPTURE?

- An acute rupture is commonly seen in squash, tennis, football, running, and other sports that require repetitive abrupt jumping or bursts of sprinting[2]

- Injury may also occur from a fall or missing a step or a deep laceration over the site of the tendon. Spontaneous ruptures during normal walking rarely occur

- The annual incidence of acute Achilles tendon rupture is around 2 in 10 000

- The incidence is rising steadily, possibly due to sedentary lifestyles and intermittent participation in recreational sport in later life[3][4]

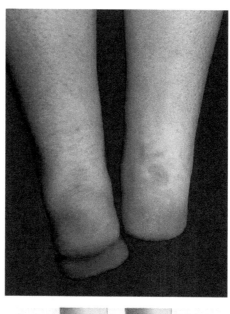

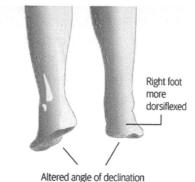

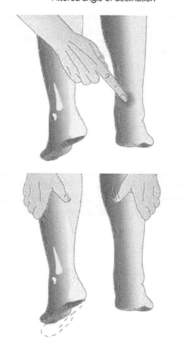

Fig 5 Compare both legs with the patient lying prone on a couch and the feet dangling over the edge. External bruising and swelling may be mild, as in this case, and relying on such signs may lead some to miss an acute rupture of the Achilles tendon. However Simmonds' triad of tests increases diagnostic accuracy. (A) Look for a difference in the angle of declination (injured right foot lies in a more dorsiflexed position). (B) Look or feel for a gap in the tendon (position of finger). (C) Squeeze the calf muscles: plantarflexion of the foot should occur if the tendon is intact (left foot), but may not occur if the tendon is ruptured (right foot)

57

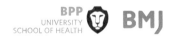

Investigations

Imaging is usually unnecessary, as the diagnosis can be made clinically. Ultrasonography or magnetic resonance imaging may help if the diagnosis is unclear (partial rupture or tendonopathy). However, when an acute Achilles rupture is suspected, it is preferable to refer the patient on the same day to an orthopaedic surgeon rather than request investigations that may delay treatment.[14]

How is it managed?

Prognosis is good with prompt treatment: normal walking and stair climbing should be possible at a median of 12 weeks after treatment, and return to sports at 9 months.[15] The goal of treatment is to restore continuity and normal length and tension of the Achilles tendon. Treatment may be surgical or non-surgical, there is no clear evidence for an optimal method.[16] Although surgery ensures a correct apposition of the tendon ends (hence a lower re-rupture rate), complications such as wound breakdown and wound infection may occur. Return to pre-injury level of activity may be achieved without surgery, especially with accelerated functional rehabilitation and early motion.[16] [17] Non-surgical management is generally best for older, less active patients or those with comorbidities. Surgical management is usually recommended for young people, athletes and people with high levels of activity, and those in whom non-surgical management has been unsuccessful. All patients, whether treated surgically or non-surgically, should have supervised physiotherapy for several months.

The risks of thromboembolic episodes[18] after acute Achilles tendon ruptures have been found to be high in some studies: discuss the risks and benefits of thrombo-prophylaxis with the patient and monitor carefully for this complication.

Competing interests: I have read and understood the BMJ Group policy on declaration of interests and have no relevant interests to declare.

Provenance and peer review: Not commissioned; externally peer reviewed.

1   Chiodo CP, Wilson MG. Current concepts review: acute ruptures of the achilles tendon. Foot Ankle Int 2006;27:305-13.
2   Jozsa L, Kvist M, Balint BJ, et al. The role of recreational sport activity in Achilles tendon rupture. A clinical, pathoanatomical, and sociological study of 292 cases. Am J Sports Med1989;17:338-43.
3   Hess GW. Achilles tendon rupture: a review of etiology, population, anatomy, risk factors, and injury prevention. Foot Ankle Spec2010;3:29-32.
4   Leppilahti J, Puranen J, Orava S. Incidence of Achilles tendon rupture. Acta Orthop Scand1996;67:277-9.
5   Inglis AE, Scott WN, Sculco TP, et al. Ruptures of the tendo achillis. An objective assessment of surgical and non-surgical treatment. J Bone Joint Surg Am1976;58:990-3.
6   MDU. Guidance and advice. Case studies: Ruptured Achilles tendon. 2010. www.themdu.com/ guidance-and-advice/case-studies/ruptured-achilles-tendon.
7   Christensen I. Rupture of the Achilles tendon: analysis of 57 cases. Acta Chir Scand1953;106:50-60.
8   Padanilam TG. Chronic Achilles tendon ruptures. Foot Ankle Clin2009;14:711-28.
9   Simmonds FA. The diagnosis of the ruptured Achilles tendon. Practitioner1957;179:56-8.
10 Thompson TC, Doherty JH. Spontaneous rupture of tendon of Achilles: a new clinical diagnostic test. J Trauma1962;2:126-9.
11 Maffulli N. The clinical diagnosis of subcutaneous tear of the Achilles tendon. A prospective study in 174 patients. Am J Sports Med 1998;26:266-70.
12 Matles AL. Rupture of the tendo Achilles: another diagnostic sign. Bull Hosp Joint Dis 1975;36:48-51.
13 Scott BW, Chalabi AA. How the Simmonds-Thompson test works. J Bone Joint Surg Br1992;74:314-5.
14 Garras DN, Raikin SM, Bhat SB, et al. MRI is unnecessary for diagnosing acute Achilles tendon ruptures: clinical diagnostic criteria. Clin Orthop Relat Res2012;470:2268-73.
15 Costa ML, MacMillan K, Halliday D, et al. Randomised controlled trials of immediate weight bearing mobilisation for rupture of the tendo Achillis. J Bone Joint Surg Br2006;88:69-77.
16 Khan RJ, Carey Smith RL. Surgical interventions for treating acute Achilles tendon ruptures. Cochrane Database Syst Rev2010;(9):CD003674.
17 Asplund CA, Best TM. Achilles tendon disorders. BMJ2013;346:f1262.
18 Makhdom AM, Cota A, Saran N, et al. Incidence of symptomatic deep venous thrombosis after Achilles tendon rupture. J Foot Ankle Surg2013;52:584-7.

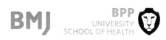

Posterior shoulder dislocations

Robert C Jacobs, resident in orthopaedic surgery,
Nicole A Meredyth, fourth year medical student,
James D Michelson, attending orthopaedic surgeon

Department of Orthopaedics and Rehabilitation, University of Vermont School of Medicine, Burlington, VT 05401, USA

Correspondence to: J D Michelson james. michelson@uvm.edu

Cite this as: BMJ 2015;350:h75

DOI: 10.1136/bmj.h75

www.bmj.com/content/350/bmj.h75

After being tackled earlier that day, a 33 year old rugby player presented to a walk in clinic with diffuse left shoulder pain, limited abduction, and arm held in slight internal rotation, with a flexed, adducted, and internally rotated position (fig 1). He was discharged and diagnosed as having a spontaneously reduced anterior shoulder dislocation after an anterioposterior view of the shoulder was read as normal (fig 2). One week later he presented to the emergency department with continued symptoms and crepitus in his shoulder with attempted movement. A posterior shoulder dislocation was diagnosed when an orthogonal view (axillary) of the shoulder was taken (fig 3). After conscious sedation, the dislocation was reduced (fig 4).

What is a posterior shoulder dislocation?

A posterior shoulder or glenohumeral dislocation is the posterior displacement of the humeral head relative to the glenoid. The anterior humeral head is typically impacted on to the glenoid rim, so patients may present with limited range of shoulder motion. Posterior shoulder dislocations are classified as acute if identified within three weeks of injury and chronic afterwards.[1] [2] Chronic posterior shoulder dislocations are often less painful and have a greater range of motion than acute posterior dislocations.[1] [3]

How common are posterior shoulder dislocations?

The glenohumeral joint is the most commonly dislocated joint in the body, and posterior shoulder dislocation comprises 2-4% of all shoulder dislocations.[4] [5] In an audit of 120 dislocations, posterior shoulder dislocations were seen most often in men aged 20-49 years, and the most common causes were traumatic events (67%) and seizures (31%).[6]

Why is it missed?

The diagnosis is often missed initially[7] [8]—delayed diagnosis occurs in 50-79% of patients.[2] [3] [9] Delay can result from the clinician or patient (or both) deeming the mechanism of injury insufficient to cause dislocation or subtle clinical examination findings relative to anterior dislocation. Patients often have enough motion in the joint and minimal palpable humeral displacement to confound a diagnosis of dislocation. Inadequate initial imaging increases the chances of missing the diagnosis. Often, only an anteroposterior view of the shoulder is ordered, without an orthogonal one; in such circumstances a posterior dislocation can look normal (fig 2).[2] [7] A dedicated protocol for shoulder injury that includes an orthogonal view significantly reduces the rate of missed diagnoses (fig 3).[6]

THE BOTTOM LINE

- Consider posterior shoulder dislocation in patients with indirect trauma and the arm flexed at the shoulder in adduction and internal rotation, or those with shoulder pain after a seizure or electrocution
- Request radiography of the shoulder with two orthogonal views, anteroposterior and axillary views being the preferred choices; however, the Velpeau or scapular Y view may also be used with the anteroposterior view
- Urgent referral to an emergency department for reduction is vital to reduce morbidity

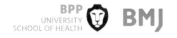

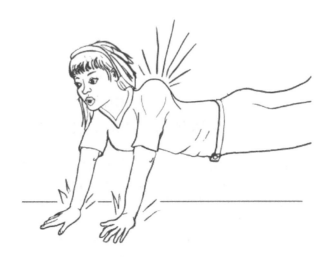

Fig 1 Diagram of mechanism of posterior dislocation: arm flexed and adducted, with internal rotation at the shoulder

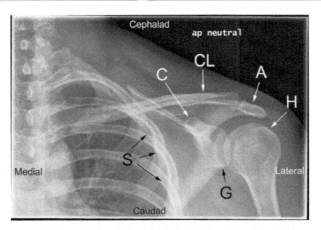

Fig 2 Pre-reduction anterioposterior radiograph of left posterior dislocation. The humeral head (H) appears to be concentrically located about the glenoid (G) and beneath the acromion (A). Slight internal rotation is present when appreciating the greater and lesser tuberosities. No fracture is seen. C=coracoid process, CL=clavicle, S=scapula

Why does it matter?

A delay in diagnosis can result in serious morbidity because posterior dislocation often produces an impression fracture on the anterior aspect of the humeral head (reverse Hill-Sachs lesion; fig 5).[4] The fracture can enlarge and propagate with prolonged dislocation while damaging the articular cartilage. This may lead to osteoarthritis and eventual avascular necrosis from impaired blood flow to the humeral head. [2 3 9 10] Early diagnosis reduces the risk of these complications and decreases the likelihood of needing a subsequent shoulder arthroplasty.[2 9]

How is it diagnosed?

Clinical diagnosis
The key to accurate and timely diagnosis is to maintain a high index of suspicion, based on mechanism of injury, and to perform appropriate diagnostic imaging. Clinical diagnosis is challenging, although specific history and physical examination findings increase the likelihood of identifying this injury. The most common mechanisms are indirect trauma, with the shoulder in a position of flexion; adduction and internal rotation, with a coaxial force applied on the arm; or extreme muscular contraction, such as seizure or electrocution.[4] Patients typically hold the affected shoulder in adduction internal rotation. They may have

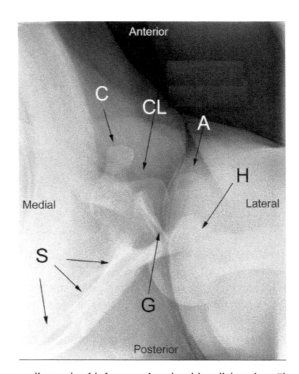

Fig 3 Pre-reduction axillary radiograph of left posterior shoulder dislocation. The humeral head (H) is clearly seen posterior and impacted on the glenoid (G). The scapular body (S) and coracoid process (C) can also be identified. The lateral aspect of the clavicle (CL) and acromion process (A) are immediately anterior to the humeral head

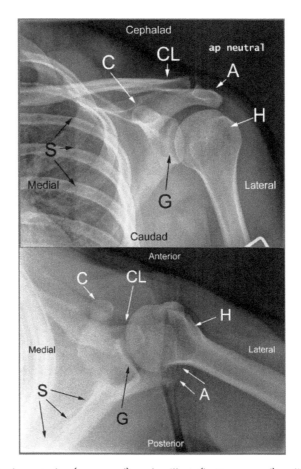

Fig 4 Post-reduction anterioposterior (top panel) and axillary (bottom panel) radiographs of the left shoulder showing concentrically located humeral head (H) within the glenoid (G). The anterioposterior views are similar before (fig 2) and after reduction, whereas the axillary views are very different (fig 3). The clavicle (CL) and acromion process (A) are superimposed on the humeral head. S=scapular body, C=coracoid process. Top of each image is anterior, bottom is posterior

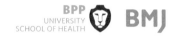

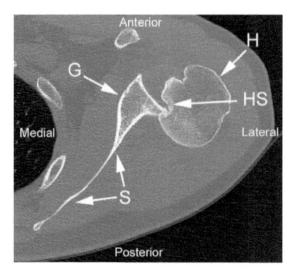

Fig 5 Pre-reduction axial computed tomogram of the left shoulder. Note the reverse Hill-Sachs impaction lesion (HS) to the anteromedial humeral head (H). G=glenoid, C=coracoid process, S=scapula

a mechanical block to external rotation, often with severe pain if the injury is acute.[6] An abnormal shoulder contour with a prominent coracoid process anteriorly and a palpable posterior positioned humeral head may be present, but the findings are often subtle.[1 4]

Posterior dislocations are often associated with other shoulder injuries, including fractures (34%), reverse Hill-Sachs injuries (29%), and rotator cuff tears (2-13%).[8]

At least two orthogonal views (anterioposterior plus axillary, Velpeau, or scapular Y) are needed to exclude a posterior dislocation.[1 7] The axillary view may require painful positioning,[3 7] and antecedent analgesia or use of a curved film cassette may help.[9] The combination of anterioposterior and Velpeau views as part of a shoulder trauma series results in an 89% detection rate of traumatic posterior shoulder dislocation.[6] Point of care ultrasound can also diagnose these injuries at the bedside, although extra training is needed and results are operator dependent.[11]

How is it managed?

Once identified, refer these dislocations to an emergency department for prompt reduction under adequate muscular relaxation. Deep procedural sedation, with airway monitoring, may be needed. Computed tomography may be needed in the emergency department to diagnose non-displaced fractures or further define fractures that could become greatly displaced with attempted closed reduction.[12] Prevention of further injury helps reduce morbidity from these injuries—many will not require operative fixation and will be able to be managed with sling immobilization.[9 12]

Thanks to Peter Weimersheimer for help in reviewing this article from the perspective of an emergency medicine physician, as well as Rachel Mauser and Nathan Mauser for their artistic contributions to figure 4B.

Contributors: RCJ and NAM searched the literature for background content on PSD and its presentation. JDM provided an orthopaedic attending perspective. All three authors helped write and revise the manuscript. JDM is guarantor.

Competing interests: We have read and understood BMJ policy on declaration of interests and have no relevant interests to declare.

Provenance and peer review: Not commissioned; externally peer reviewed.

Patient consent not required (patient anonymised, dead, or hypothetical).

1 Detenbeck LC. Posterior dislocations of the shoulder. *J Trauma* 1972;12:183-92.
2 Rowe CR, Zarins B. Chronic unreduced dislocations of the shoulder. *J Bone Joint Surg Am* 1982;64:494-505.
3 Robinson CM, Aderinto J. Posterior shoulder dislocations and fracture-dislocations. *J Bone Joint Surg Am* 2005;87-A:639-50.
4 McLaughlin HL. Posterior dislocation of the shoulder. *J Bone Joint Surg Am* 1952;24-A-3:584-90.
5 Rowe CR. Prognosis in dislocations of the shoulder. *J Bone Joint Surg Am* 1956;38-A:957-77.

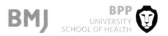

6   Robinson CM, Seah M, Akhtar MA. The epidemiology, risk of recurrence, and functional outcome after an acute traumatic posterior dislocation of the shoulder. *J Bone Joint Surg Am* 2011;93:1605-13.

7   Espag MP, Back DL, Baroni M, Bennett AR, Peckham TJ. Diagnosing shoulder dislocations: time for a change of view. *Ann R Coll Surg Engl* 2002;84:334-7.

8   Rouleau DM, Hebert-Davies J. Incidence of associated injury in posterior shoulder dislocation: systematic review of the literature. *J Orthop Trauma* 2012;26:246-51.

9   Schliemann B, Muder D, Gessmann J, Schildhauer TA, Seybold D. Locked posterior shoulder dislocation: treatment options and clinical outcomes. *Arch Orthop Trauma Surg* 2011;131:1127-34.

10 Ogawa K, Yoshida A, Inokuchi W. Posterior shoulder dislocation associated with fracture of the humeral anatomic neck: treatment guidelines and long-term outcome. *J Trauma* 1999;46:318-23.

11 Mackenzie DC, Liebmann O. Point-of-care ultrasound facilitates diagnosing a posterior shoulder dislocation. *J Emerg Med* 2013;44:976-8.

12 Rouleau DM, Hebert-Davies J, Robinson CM. Acute traumatic posterior shoulder dislocation. *J Am Acad Orthop Surg* 2014;22:145-52.

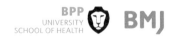

Late onset type 1 diabetes

Daniel Lasserson, senior clinical researcher[1],
Robin Fox, general practitioner[2],
Andrew Farmer, professor of general practice[1]

[1]University of Oxford, Department of Primary Care Health Sciences, Oxford OX1 2ET, UK

[2]The Health Centre, Bicester, UK

Correspondence to: D Lasserson daniel.lasserson@phc.ox.ac.uk

Cite this as: BMJ 2012;344:e2827

DOI: 10.1136/bmj.e2827

www.bmj.com/content/344/bmj.e2827

A 41 year old man from an Indian family whose father had type 2 diabetes presented to his general practitioner with a four week history of increasing thirst and polyuria. He had not noticed any weight loss. Blood tests were arranged to confirm the diagnosis of diabetes. One week later, after having to push his car home, he began to feel exhausted and developed intermittent vomiting, which he attributed to exertion. Over the next two days he became more unwell, and the out of hours primary care service was contacted. He was reviewed urgently and admitted with diabetic ketoacidosis.

What is late onset type 1 diabetes?

A spectrum of autoimmune diabetes presents in adulthood, with type 1 diabetes characterised by the requirement of insulin at diagnosis to control glycaemia and prevent ketogenesis. Latent autoimmune diabetes of adulthood (LADA) also occurs but with much slower progression to requiring insulin after initial diagnosis.

Why is it missed?

Similar rates of ketoacidosis are seen in patients with type 1 diabetes at diagnosis in adulthood and childhood,[3] and diagnostic delay is thought to account for many presentations with ketoacidosis in children.[4] Although the classic symptoms produced by hyperglycaemia are unlikely to be missed, there may be a delay in accurately identifying patients requiring insulin at diagnosis if there is a clinical resemblance to type 2 diabetes at initial consultation. Family history is an important component of diagnostic reasoning in primary care, and, although type 2 diabetes has a strong familial link, the incidence of type 1 diabetes is also increased in relatives of patients with type 2 diabetes.[5]

Why does this matter?

Delay in diagnosis of type 1 diabetes can result in the development of ketoacidosis, requiring intensive management in secondary care. Patients may also be unnecessarily exposed to the risks from dehydration, acidosis, potassium shifts, and renal failure. Large cohort studies of patients with type 1 diabetes show that, although long term health has improved substantially for those with disease of childhood onset, this has not been the case for those with onset during adulthood,[6] and mortality during the first two years after diagnosis is also higher in adult onset type 1 diabetes compared with childhood onset.[7]

KEY POINTS

- Delay in diagnosis of adult onset type 1 diabetes can result in progression to ketoacidosis
- Some families have a mix of type 1 and type 2 diabetes in their pedigrees, so family history is an unreliable guide for classifying type of diabetes
- Routinely test for ketonuria on suspicion of diabetes in adults even if there is convincing evidence for type 2 diabetes
- When making a diagnosis of type 2 diabetes in a young adult in primary care, ensure that the patient is aware of the symptoms of progression to ketoacidosis to prompt early healthcare contact for reassessment

---

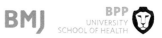

HOW COMMON IS LATE ONSET TYPE 1 DIABETES?

- In the 30–50 year age group, type 1 diabetes accounts for 13% of all new cases of diabetes[1]

- Annual incidence is 15/100000 in the 15–34 year age group, increasing by 2.8% annually,[2] and is 7/100000 in the 30–50 age group[1]

How is type 1 diabetes diagnosed in adults?

Clinical features

A small cohort study reported that the classic symptoms of hyperglycaemia (thirst and polyuria) were observed at diagnosis of both adult and childhood onset type 1 diabetes, but the time course of symptoms was longer in adults (five weeks compared with two weeks) with less weight loss and few preceding superficial infections in the prodromal stage.[3] In type 2 diabetes the prodrome of symptoms of hyperglycaemia can be longer, with 20% of patients symptomatic for up to six months before diagnosis.[8] The symptoms and time course of type 1 diabetes can therefore overlap with those of type 2 diabetes, and there are no reliable clinical predictors from history and physical examination that will distinguish type 1 from type 2 diabetes in young adults. However, the National Institute for Health and Clinical Excellence (NICE) recommends that type 1 diabetes should be suspected if there is weight loss or lack of features of the metabolic syndrome in someone with newly diagnosed diabetes.[9]

If diabetic ketoacidosis has developed, common features are lethargy and vomiting with an increased respiratory rate and tachycardia, and in severe presentations, reduced level of consciousness, deep sighing respiration, and collapse.

Investigations

With new onset diabetes in young adults, the traditional categories of type 1 (insulin requiring) and type 2 (insulin resistant), which are oversimplifications, are not easily discriminated at initial presentation.[10] The diagnostic criteria for diabetes, irrespective of type, are more straightforward, with random plasma glucose concentration $\geq$11.1 mmol/L and fasting plasma glucose concentration $\geq$7.0 mmol/L (in the presence of symptoms only one of these criteria is required).[9] Diagnosis by means of HbA1c is not recommended for type 1 diabetes.

Although a large prospective cohort study showed that type 1 and type 2 diabetes can be differentiated using laboratory markers for aetiology and level of insulin secretion (autoantibodies and C peptide levels),[11] they are not yet recommended for routine use in supporting diagnosis.

NICE recommends initial assessment for ketonuria as a marker of the need for exogenous insulin[9] as other routinely ordered tests are unlikely to alert the clinician to the possibility of type 1 diabetes. Cohort studies based in secondary care show that up to 20% of patients with adult onset type 1 diabetes do not have ketonuria at presentation.[3] However, there are no community based studies of late onset type 1 diabetes, so the prevalence of ketonuria at initial presentation in primary care is not known. Nevertheless, continuing review and reassessment may be needed when the initial diagnosis is unclear, particularly if there is rapid clinical deterioration.[10] Making all patients with newly diagnosed diabetes in primary care aware of the symptoms of progression to ketoacidosis may prompt earlier healthcare contact for the minority who have type 1 diabetes that is initially misclassified as type 2.

How is late onset type 1 diabetes managed?

Initiate insulin at diagnosis to control blood glucose levels and suppress ketogenesis. Most patients will require acute assessment in secondary care for renal function, acid-base balance, and ketone body levels, as these will guide the need for intravenous therapy with insulin, fluid, and electrolytes. Detect and manage any underlying precipitants such as infection.

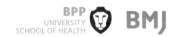

After initial stabilisation, a number of different insulin regimens may be suitable depending on agreed goals of therapy, although optimal glucose control requires long acting insulin to suppress fasting glucose levels and short acting insulin to reduce postprandial levels. Offer structured education encompassing dietary and lifestyle advice, self monitoring of blood glucose with adjustment of insulin doses, insulin treatment during periods of illness, and complications of diabetes. Undertake vascular risk assessment to identify and control risk factors with additional treatment. Coordination between primary and secondary care is essential to provide effective long term support.

All authors contributed to reviewing relevant evidence and writing the manuscript. DSL is guarantor.

All authors have completed the Unified Competing Interest form at www.icmje.org/coi_disclosure.pdf (available on request from the corresponding author) and declare: no support from any organisation for the submitted work; no financial relationships with any organisations that might have an interest in the submitted work in the previous three years, no other relationships or activities that could appear to have influenced the submitted work.

Provenance and peer review: Commissioned and externally peer reviewed.

Patient consent obtained.

1   Bruno G, Runzo C, Cavallo-Perin P, Merletti F, Rivetti M, Pinach S, et al. Incidence of type 1 and type 2 diabetes in adults aged 30-49 years: the population-based registry in the province of Turin, Italy. *Diabetes Care* 2005;28:2613-9.
2   Imkampe AK, Gulliford MC. Trends in type 1 diabetes incidence in the UK in 0- to 14-year-olds and in 15- to 34-year-olds, 1991-2008. *Diabet Med* 2011;28:811-4.
3   Sabbah E, Savola K, Ebeling T, Kulmala P, Vahasalo P, Ilonen J, et al. Genetic, autoimmune, and clinical characteristics of childhood- and adult-onset type 1 diabetes. *Diabetes Care* 2000;23:1326-32.
4   Usher-Smith JA, Thompson MJ, Sharp SJ, Walter FM. Factors associated with the presence of diabetic ketoacidosis at diagnosis of diabetes in children and young adults: a systematic review. *BMJ* 2011;343:d4092.
5   Tuomi T. Type 1 and type 2 diabetes: what do they have in common? *Diabetes* 2005;54(suppl 2):S40-5.
6   Harjutsalo V, Forsblom C, Groop PH. Time trends in mortality in patients with type 1 diabetes: nationwide population based cohort study. *BMJ* 2011;343:d5364.
7   Bruno G, Cerutti F, Merletti F, Novelli G, Panero F, Zucco C, et al. Short-term mortality risk in children and young adults with type 1 diabetes: the population-based registry of the province of Turin, Italy. *Nutr Metab Cardiovasc Dis* 2009;19:340-4.
8   Drivsholm T, de Fine ON, Nielsen AB, Siersma V. Symptoms, signs and complications in newly diagnosed type 2 diabetic patients, and their relationship to glycaemia, blood pressure and weight. *Diabetologia* 2005;48:210-4.
9   National Collaborating Centre for Women's and Children's Health, National Collaborating Centre for Chronic Conditions. *Type 1 diabetes: diagnosis and management of type 1 diabetes in children, young people and adults* . National Institute for Health and Clinical Excellence, 2004.
10 Royal College of General Practitioners, NHS Diabetes. Coding, classification and diagnosis of diabetes. 2011. www.diabetes.nhs.uk/our_work_areas/classification_of_diabetes/.
11 Zimmet P, Turner R, McCarty D, Rowley M, Mackay I. Crucial points at diagnosis. Type 2 diabetes or slow type 1 diabetes. *Diabetes Care* 1999;22(suppl 2):B59-64.

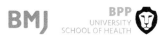

Acute Charcot foot

Piero Baglioni, physician in endocrinology and diabetes[1],
Manzar Malik, consultant radiologist[2],
Onyebuchi E Okosieme, consultant physician in endocrinology and diabetes[1]

[1]Department of Endocrinology and Diabetes, Prince Charles Hospital, Cwm Taf Local Health Board, Merthyr Tydfil CF47 9DT, UK

[2]Department of Radiology, Prince Charles Hospital

Correspondence to: O E Okosieme Onyebuchi. Okosieme@Wales.nhs.uk

Cite this as: BMJ 2012;344:e1397

DOI: 10.1136/bmj.e1397

www.bmj.com/content/344/bmj.e1397

A 38 year old man was referred by his general practitioner to our diabetes foot clinic with a swollen red foot (fig 1). He had had type 1 diabetes for 25 years, complicated with retinopathy, peripheral neuropathy, and nephropathy, and was being worked up for dialysis following a failed pancreas-kidney transplant. The absence of pain together with preserved pulses and intact skin raised a suspicion of acute Charcot foot. A plain radiograph of the foot showed fractures through the necks of the first three metatarsals (fig 2). We offloaded the foot in a total contact cast and advised the patient to limit weight bearing. Magnetic resonance imaging (MRI) subsequently confirmed neuroarthropathic changes of acute Charcot (fig 3).

What is acute Charcot foot?

Charcot's neuroarthropathy is a destructive process of bone and joint, typically seen in a foot that has lost its protective sensory innervation. The classic description of this disabling condition by Jean-Martin Charcot in 1883 was in patients with tabes dorsalis, but nowadays most cases of Charcot foot occur as a complication of diabetes mellitus. The chronic stage of the disease is easily recognisable, but the acute phase can present a diagnostic challenge.[1] In a recent series the diagnosis of acute Charcot foot was missed before specialist referral in 19 of 20 patients.[2] In another report, referring clinicians failed to diagnose Charcot foot in 19 of 24 cases seen in a specialist diabetes foot clinic.[3]

Why is acute Charcot foot missed?

The acute phase of a Charcot foot may not be considered or may be mistaken for more common causes of leg or foot swelling, such as cellulitis, gout, deep venous thrombosis, or sprains.[2] The misdiagnosis of ankle sprain is particularly common if the patient recalls a history of trivial injury. Standard radiographs may show no abnormalities at this stage, contributing to delays in diagnosis.[3]

Why does this matter?

The delay in correct diagnosis is harmful because during the acute phase the foot bones are vulnerable to fragmentation and dislocation.[1] If the patient continues to walk on an insensitive foot, this may lead—sometimes within weeks—to irreversible deformities, such as mid-foot dislocation or collapse and inversion of the plantar arch, the so called rocker-bottom foot. These deformities may, in turn, predispose to skin ulcer, an established risk factor for amputation.[4] If the disease is diagnosed in the acute phase, bone and joint damage can largely be prevented by avoiding weight bearing.[1] Timely recognition may also

---

KEY POINTS

- Suspect acute Charcot foot in a patient with diabetes and neuropathy who presents with a swollen warm foot
- If acute Charcot foot is suspected, arrange for offloading of the foot (to minimise further damage) and refer to a specialist foot clinic immediately
- Plain radiographs may be normal in the early stages of the disease
- Magnetic resonance imaging should be considered when the suspicion of acute Charcot foot is high

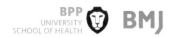

HOW COMMON IS ACUTE CHARCOT FOOT?

- The true incidence of acute Charcot foot is difficult to establish, because few population based studies have been published and no diagnostic criteria have been universally agreed

- The reported annual incidence of Charcot arthropathy in patients with diabetes has varied from 0.3% in population studies[11] to 12.0% in referral centre studies[7]

- Studies in specialist units report that Charcot arthropathy was present in 9% of patients with diabetic neuropathy and foot ulcer[12] and in 12% of diabetic patients who had received pancreas-kidney transplants[7]

---

identify patients with diabetes who are at increased risk of mortality owing to the severe neuropathy associated with Charcot foot.[5] In one series, patients with acute Charcot foot or neuropathic foot ulcers had a 5-year mortality rate of 40%.[5] Mortality may relate to co-existent renal disease in some patients, but neuropathy is also believed to independently increase cardiovascular risk by promoting vascular calcification.[6]

How is acute Charcot foot diagnosed?

Clinical features

The usual presentation is a red, swollen, warm foot in which pulses are preserved (fig 1). Owing to neuropathy, pain is not always present or is less than expected for the severity of the clinical findings. Longstanding diabetes, either type 1 or type 2, or a history of renal transplantation confer a particularly high risk.[7] The patient may be thought at this stage to have gout, ankle sprain, or deep venous thrombosis, but the most common misdiagnosis is infection. The presence of an ulcer favours the diagnosis of cellulitis or osteomyelitis, particularly if this can be probed to bone. Absence of skin break, stable insulin requirements, and normal white blood cell counts or C-reactive protein levels are more suggestive of acute Charcot than infection.[8] Neuro-arthropathy and infection are, however, not mutually exclusive and if any doubt exists the patient should be treated for both conditions until the true diagnosis is established.[8]

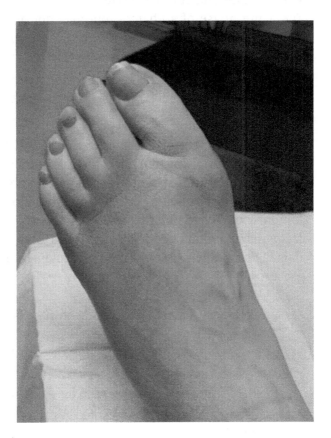

Fig 1 Acute Charcot foot

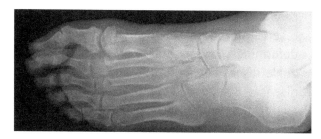

Fig 2 Plain radiograph of the foot showing fractures through the necks of the first three metatarsals

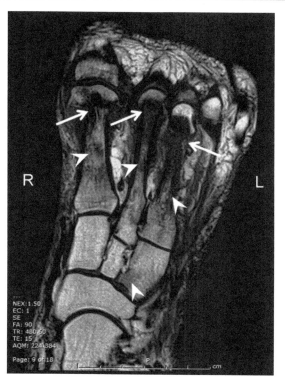

Fig 3 Axial T1 weighted MRI showing pathological fractures through the necks of the first three metatarsals (arrows) with oedema in metatarsal shafts and lateral cuneiform bones (arrow heads). These features, in a patient with diabetes and no history of trauma, suggest acute Charcot foot

Investigations

Standard radiographs are an important first line investigation. The finding of fractures or bony misalignment in the absence of obvious trauma is highly suggestive of Charcot foot (fig 2). The initial radiograph may be normal, but this should not divert from the diagnosis if the clinical suspicion is high.[3] A radioisotope bone scan or MRI can show bone disease even when radiographic changes are subtle (fig 3). The choice between nuclear imaging and MRI is largely based on local availability and experience.[9] Bone scan has less specificity than MRI (25-38% v 80-100%), but the diagnostic sensitivity of either test approaches 100%.[10] The mid-foot region is the most common site of disease, although hind-foot involvement carries a particularly severe prognosis owing to the risk of ankle instability. MRI is the investigation of choice in patients with ulcers and a high probability of deep infection. However, the differentiation of Charcot from osteomyelitis may occasionally be difficult even with MRI.[9] [10]

How is acute Charcot foot managed?

If acute Charcot foot is suspected, seek urgent referral to a specialist foot clinic and advise patients to avoid weight bearing pending evaluation[8] Early offloading of the foot with total contact casting is the gold standard of treatment.[9] Casting is usually needed for three to six months, and healing is indicated by resolution of oedema and warmth. Radiographic or MRI evidence of healing assists the clinical decision to discontinue casting and transfer the patient into a bespoke shoe.[9] A lifelong programme of patient education and routine foot

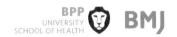

care should form an essential component of treatment. Reconstructive surgery is currently reserved for patients in whom attempts at conservative care have failed to prevent major deformities. Earlier surgical intervention could nonetheless be considered for patients with ankle disease owing to the often limited success of conservative measures in this form of disease.[9] Bisphosphonates have been proposed to counteract the excess bone turnover that characterises the acute Charcot foot, but the evidence for their benefit is still inconclusive.[9]

Contributors: PB had the original idea for the paper and wrote the first draft of the paper. All authors contributed to the planning, drafting, and revision of the paper and all approved the final version of the paper. OEO is the guarantor.

Competing interests: All authors have completed the Unified Competing Interest form at www.icmje. org/coi_disclosure.pdf (available on request from the corresponding author) and declare: no support from any organisation for the submitted work; no financial relationships with any organisations that might have an interest in the submitted work in the previous three years; no other relationships or activities that could appear to have influenced the submitted work.

Provenance and peer review: Not commissioned; externally peer reviewed.

Patient consent obtained.

1   Hartemann-Heurtier A, Van GH, Grimaldi A. The Charcot foot. *Lancet* 2002;360:1776-9.
2   Wukich DK, Sung W, Wipf SA, Armstrong DG. The consequences of complacency: managing the effects of unrecognized Charcot feet. *Diabet Med* 2011;28:195-8.
3   Chantelau E. The perils of procrastination: effects of early vs delayed detection and treatment of incipient Charcot fracture. *Diabet Med* 2005;22:1707-12.
4   Sohn MW, Stuck RM, Pinzur M, Lee TA, Budiman-Mak E. Lower-extremity amputation risk after charcot arthropathy and diabetic foot ulcer. *Diabetes Care* 2010;33:98-100.
5   Van Baal J, Hubbard R, Game F, Jeffcoate W. Mortality associated with acute Charcot foot and neuropathic foot ulceration. *Diabetes Care* 2010;33:1086-9.
6   Jeffcoate WJ, Rasmussen LM, Hofbauer LC, Game FL. Medial arterial calcification in diabetes and its relationship to neuropathy. *Diabetologia* 2009;52:2478-88.
7   Matricali GA, Bammens B, Kuypers D, Flour M, Mathieu C. High rate of Charcot foot attacks early after simultaneous pancreas-kidney transplantation. *Transplantation* 2007;83:245-6.
8   Edmonds M, Foster AVM, Sanders LJ. Charcot foot. In: A practical manual of diabetic foot care. 2nd ed. Blackwell Publishing, 2008:63-78
9   Rogers LC, Frykberg RG, Armstrong DG, Boulton AJ, Edmonds M, Van GH, et al. The Charcot foot in diabetes. *Diabetes Care* 2011;34:2123-9.
10 Rogers LC, Bevilacqua NJ. Imaging of the Charcot foot. *Clin Podiatr Med Surg* 2008;25:263-74.
11 Fabrin J, Larsen K, Holstein PE. Long-term follow-up in diabetic Charcot feet with spontaneous onset. *Diabetes Care* 2000;23:796-800.
12 Cavanagh PR, Young MJ, Adams JE, Vickers KL, Boulton AJ. Radiographic abnormalities in the feet of patients with diabetic neuropathy. *Diabetes Care* 1994;17:201-9.

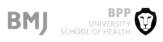
Subdural haematoma in the elderly

Elizabeth A Teale, clinical senior lecturer[1],
Steve Iliffe, professor of primary care for older people[2],
John B Young, professor of elderly care medicine[1]

[1]Academic Unit for Elderly Care and Rehabilitation, Leeds Institute of Health Sciences, Bradford BD9 6RJ, UK

[2]Department of Primary Care and Population Health, University College London, London NW3 2PF, UK

Correspondence to: E A Teale Elizabeth.Teale@bthft.nhs.uk

Cite this as: *BMJ* 2014;348:g1682

DOI: 10.1136/bmj.g1682

www.bmj.com/content/348/bmj.g1682

An 84 year old woman with a history of postural hypotension and frequent falls presented with a two week history of confusion and wandering. Her general practitioner diagnosed delirium secondary to a urinary tract infection on the basis of a positive urinary dipstick test for white blood cells and nitrites. She failed to improve with oral antibiotics and was admitted to hospital for further assessment. Clinical examination showed a lack of focal neurological signs but cranial computed tomography revealed a left sided chronic subdural haematoma.

What is a subdural haematoma?

A subdural haematoma results from tearing of the veins linking the cerebral cortex and the dural sinuses, causing blood to accumulate between the dura and arachnoid maters. Brain atrophy associated with ageing or dementia stretches these fragile veins such that they are more prone to tearing after relatively trivial (and often forgotten) head injury[1]; in up to half of cases there is a history of fall without head trauma.[1 2 3] Over time, there is fibrin deposition and organisation of the haematoma, resulting in a chronic subdural haematoma. Neovascularisation processes within the subdural haematoma increase the propensity for acute or chronic bleeding.[4] Anticoagulation increases the risk of subdural haematoma and the likelihood of fresh bleeding into an established haematoma.[4]

Why is it missed?

Only about half of people presenting with a subdural haematoma give a history of a direct head trauma or a fall with a head injury. A fall without head injury may account for a further 33-54% of cases.[3 5] There may be a long delay between the fall or trauma and the onset of symptoms (mean 49 days, range 15 to 751 days).[10] Cranial imaging performed shortly after a fall or head trauma can be normal in individuals who go on to develop a chronic subdural haematoma and may falsely reassure.[11 12]

The clinical features of a subdural haematoma can easily be misinterpreted. Subdural haematoma can mimic alcohol excess.[13] A presentation with behavioural or personality changes may be mistaken for a psychiatric disorder[14 15] or dementia,[16] especially in patients where these conditions pre-exist.[14] Delirium (acute confusion) is a common feature of subdural haematoma, especially in older people (52% of 56 patients aged >60 with subdural haematoma in one case series),[17] and may be falsely ascribed to other, more common causes of delirium such as infections or medicines. Transient neurological deficits are the presenting feature in 1-21% of chronic subdural haematomas,[1 2 5] leading to the potential for a mistaken diagnosis of transient ischaemic attack.[18]

KEY POINTS

- Many patients with a confirmed subdural haematoma have no history of fall or head injury
- Chronic subdural haematomas can present with confusion, behavioural or personality changes, or neurological features that may be mistaken for delirium falsely ascribed to another cause (such as infection), psychiatric illness, or transient ischaemic attack
- The absence of neurological signs does not exclude the possibility of a chronic subdural haematoma
- The diagnosis of a chronic subdural haematoma is made by non-contrast cranial computed tomography (CT) imaging

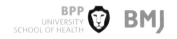

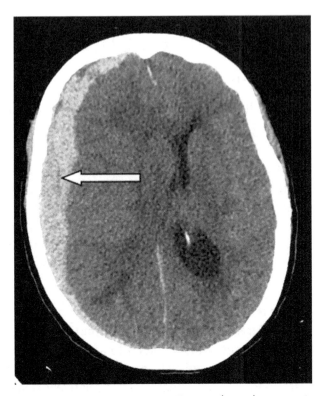

Fig 1 Crescentic right side high attenuation subdural collection (arrow), suggesting acute subdural haematoma. There is substantial mass effect and oedema with effacement of the ventricle and midline shift

In patients presenting to hospital with a subdural haematoma, two case series found that the diagnosis was not suspected before imaging in 62-80% of cases.[2] [5]

Why does this matter?

There is evidence that cognitive, gait, behavioural, focal neurological, extra-pyramidal, and psychiatric disturbances can improve or be reversed following neurosurgical intervention to treat a chronic subdural haematoma.[4] [14] [16] [19] [20] [21] Continued expansion of a chronic subdural haematoma, or fresh bleeding into an established haematoma, can result in deterioration, over hours, days, or weeks that may result in persistent neurological deficit[13] or death.

HOW COMMON IS SUBDURAL HAEMATOMA?

- The incidence of chronic subdural haematoma increases with age[1]

- Case series data from 1996 to 1999 estimate the incidence of chronic subdural haematoma in over 65 year olds at 8.2/100000/year.[5] A recent retrospective case series study from Japan reports the incidence of chronic subdural haematoma in older people to be 76.5/100000/year in 70-79 year olds and 127/100000/year in those aged .80.[6] These higher estimates may reflect better access to diagnostic imaging

- Two high quality randomised controlled trials estimate absolute rates of chronic subdural haematoma for patients aged >75 years taking warfarin as 0.2-0.31% per annum[7] [8]

- In a large randomised controlled trial, dabigatran was associated with a lower absolute risk of subdural haematoma than warfarin for patients with atrial fibrillation. This seemed to be dose dependent (absolute annual risk of subdural haematoma with warfarin 0.31%, with 110 mg twice daily dabigatran 0.08%, with 150 mg twice daily dabigatran 0.20%)[7]

- A recent meta-analysis of published and unpublished data from nine randomised controlled trials did not find a statistically significant association between aspirin therapy and subdural haematoma (odds ratio 1.6 (95% confidence interval 0.8 to 3.5) v placebo)[9]

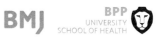

How is subdural haematoma diagnosed?

Clinical features

Consider the diagnosis of chronic subdural haematoma as cause or consequence of new onset falls or increased fall frequency (74% in one series[2]). Other common features are behavioural or cognitive disturbances (present in 34-55% of patients)[1 5 10 22] and transient (1-21% of patients), persistent or progressive focal neurological deficits (24% to 88% of patients).[1 2 5 10 22] Headache is the presenting feature in 14-27% of patients,[2 5 10 22] reduced consciousness is present in 2.9-35%,[2 5 22] and a seizure is the presenting event for 10-14%.[2 10] Features of raised intracranial pressure such as nausea, vomiting, headache, or altered consciousness and neurological features are less common in older people because brain atrophy provides space to accommodate the haematoma. The indolent course of chronic subdural haematoma should prompt reconsideration of the diagnosis in the presence of persistent symptoms, neurological deficit, or features of raised intracranial pressure even if initial imaging is normal.

There should be a particularly high index of suspicion for a diagnosis of subdural haematoma in patients treated with anticoagulant drugs. Case series have reported that 9-21% of patients presenting with subdural haematomas are treated with anticoagulants.[10 23 24 25] The absolute annual risk of subdural haematoma in patients taking warfarin has been estimated at 0.2% with a therapeutic international normalised ratio (INR) of 2-3,[8] and risk increases substantially with a supratherapeutic INR.[26] A large randomised controlled trial has shown that, compared with warfarin, dabigatran is associated with a lower absolute risk of subdural haematoma (see box "How common is subdural haematoma?").[7] Onset of symptoms in patients treated with anticoagulants is generally more rapid than in the general population (80% present within a week[26]), and features of raised intracranial pressure or focal neurological deficit are prominent (headache, nausea and vomiting, reduced consciousness, hemiparesis, ataxia),[26] even in older people.

Investigations

The diagnosis of a subdural haematoma is made by non-contrast cranial computed tomography. The clot appears as a crescent shaped opacity around the cerebral hemisphere (see figure).[4] An acute subdural haematoma appears as a hyperdense lesion. As the subdural haematoma matures, there is transition through isodensity to the hypodense appearance of a chronic subdural haematoma.[27] Features of midline shift may help to alert to the presence of unilateral subdural haematoma in the isodense phase,[27] but in bilateral chronic subdural haematomas (16-20% of cases[28]) where midline shift may not be apparent, more subtle radiological features such as effacement of the sulci suggest the diagnosis.[27 28] A high index of clinical suspicion is therefore required reliably to interpret the CT scan findings.

How is subdural haematoma managed?

Rapid reversal of anticoagulants and discontinuation of antiplatelet therapy are required for patients presenting with a subdural haematoma on these medications. Small subdural haematomas that are asymptomatic and without radiological features of raised intracranial pressure may be managed conservatively[4] with follow-up by clinical assessment and repeat CT scanning if deterioration is apparent. However, if there is neurological compromise, or features of brain compression on imaging, evacuation of the clot via craniostomy (drilling a hole through the skull) or craniotomy (where a piece of the skull is removed and then replaced) is indicated.[4] Older patients with large haematomas and midline shift have particularly poor outcomes, particularly without surgical intervention.[2 10]

We thank Dr Samad Punekar for help in preparing the image.

Contributors: ET and JY searched the literature for background content on SDH and its presentation. SI provided a primary care perspective. All authors contributed to drafting and revising the manuscript. JY acts as guarantor.

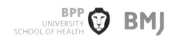

Competing interests: We have read and understood the BMJ Group policy on declaration of interests and have no relevant interests to declare.

Provenance and peer review: Commissioned; externally peer reviewed.

Consent obtained from a relative.

1   Adhiyaman V, Asghar M, Ganeshram KN, Bhowmick BK. Chronic subdural haematoma in the elderly. *Postgrad Med J* 2002;78:71-5.
2   Jones S, Kafetz K. A propective study of chronic subdural haematomas in elderly patients. *Age Ageing* 1999;28:519-21.
3   Rozzelle CJ, Wofford JL, Branch CL. Predictors of hospital mortality in older patients with subdural hematoma. *J Am Geriatr Soc* 1995;43:240-4.
4   Ducruet AF, Grobelny BT, Zacharia BE, Hickman ZL, DeRosa PL, Anderson K, et al. The surgical management of chronic subdural haematoma. *Neurosurg Rev* 2011;35:155-69.
5   Asghar M, Adhiyaman V, Greenway M, Bhowmick B, Bates A. Chronic subdural haematoma in the elderly—a North Wales experience. *J R Soc Med* 2002;95:290-2.
6   Karibe H, Kameyama M, Kawase M, Hirano T, Kawaguchi T, Tominaga T. [Epidemiology of chronic subdural hematomas] (Japanese). *No Shinkei Geka* 2011;39:1149-53.
7   Hart RG, Diener H-C, Yang S, Connolly SJ, Wallentin L, Reilly PA, et al. Intracranial hemorrhage in atrial fibrillation patients during anticoagulation with warfarin or dabigatran: the RE-LY trial. *Stroke* 2012;43:1511-7.
8   Mant J, Hobbs R, Fletcher K, Roalfe A, Fitzmaurice D, Lip G, et al. Warfarin versus aspirin for stroke prevention in an elderly community population with atrial fibrillation (the Birmingham Atrial Fibrillation Treatment of the Aged Study, BAFTA): a randomised controlled trial. *Lancet* 2007;370:493-503.
9   Connolly BJ, Pearce LA, Kurth T, Kase CS, Hart RG. Aspirin therapy and risk of subdural hematoma: meta-analysis of randomized clinical trials. *J Stroke Cerebrovasc Dis* 2013;22:444-8
10 Gelabert-González M, Iglesias-Pais M, García-Allut A, Martínez-Rumbo R. Chronic subdural haematoma: surgical treatment and outcome in 1000 cases. *Clin Neurol Neurosurg* 2005;107:223-9.
11 Medical Protection Society. An evolving situation. *Casebook* 2010;18:17.
12 Snoey ER, Levitt MA. Delayed diagnosis of subdural hematoma following normal computed tomography scan. *Ann Emerg Med* 1994;23:1127-31.
13 Medical Protection Society. Case 4: cerebrally impaired or just drunk? *UK Casebook* 2003;11:10.
14 Henderson M. A difficult psychiatric patient. *Postgrad Med J* 2000;76:585-6.
15 Singh TB, Devi AR, Singh SG, Bhagwan MB. Chronic subdural haematoma presenting as late onset psychosis. *ASEAN J Psychiatry* 2013;14:175-8.
16 Ishikawa E, Yanaka K, Sugimoto K. Reversible dementia in patients with chronic subdural hematomas. *J Neurosurg* 2002;96:680-3.
17 Black DW. Mental changes resulting from subdural haematoma. *Br J Psychiatry* 1984;145:200-3.
18 Guptha SH, Puthrasingam S. A case of chronic subdural haematoma presenting as a transient ischaemic attack. *Age Ageing* 2001;30:172-3.
19 Bostanjopoulou S, Katsarou Z, Michael M, Petridis A. Reversible parkinsonism due to chronic bilateral subdural hematomas. *J Clin Neurosci* 2009;16;458-460.
20 Crandon IW, Eldemire-Shearer D, Fearon Boothe D, Morris C, James K. A case report of chronic subdural haematomas in two elderly patients. *West Indian Med J* 2007;56:547-9.
21 Velasco J, Head M, Farlin E, Lippmann S. Unsuspected subdural hematoma as a differential diagnosis in elderly patients. *South Med J* 1995;88:977-9.
22 Liliang P, Tsai Y, Liang C, Lee T, Chen H. Chronic subdural haematoma in young and extremely aged adults: a comparative study of two age groups. *Injury* 2002;33:345-8.
23 Aspegren OP, Astrand R, Lundgren MI, Romner B. Anticoagulation therapy a risk factor for the development of chronic subdural hematoma. *Clin Neurol Neurosurg* 2013;115:981-4.
24 Jeffree RL, Gordon DH, Sivasubramaniam R, Chapman A. Warfarin related intracranial haemorrhage: a case-controlled study of anticoagulation monitoring prior to spontaneous subdural or intracerebral haemorrhage. *J Fam Pract* 2009;16:882-5.
25 Rust T, Kiemer N, Erasmus A. Chronic subdural haematomas and anticoagulation or anti-thrombotic therapy. *J Fam Pract* 2006;13:823-7.
26 Hylek EM, Singer DE. Risk factors for intracranial hemorrhage in outpatients taking warfarin. *Ann Intern Med* 1994;120:897-902.
27 Davenport RJ, Statham PF, Warlow CP. Detection of bilateral isodense dubdural haematomas. *BMJ* 1994;309:792-4.
28 Sadrolhefazi AA, Bloomfield SMS. Interhemishperic and bilateral chronic subdural hematoma. *Neurosurg Clin N Am* 2000;11:455-63.

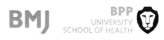

Myasthenia gravis

J Spillane, clinical research associate[1],
E Higham, general practitioner partner[2],
D M Kullmann, professor of neurology[1]

[1]UCL Institute of
Neurology, London
WC1N3BG, UK

[2]Central Medical Centre,
Morden SM4 5RT, UK

Correspondence to:
J Spillane jennifer.
spillane.09@ucl.ac.uk

Cite this as: BMJ
2012;345:e8497

DOI: 10.1136/bmj.e8497

www.bmj.com/
content/345/bmj.e8497

A previously well 78 year old man presented to his general practitioner with a six month history of double vision that was more pronounced when he was tired. His wife had also noted drooping of his eyelids towards the end of the day. Examination showed restricted eye movements (ophthalmoplegia) and fatigable ptosis. He was referred to his local neurology centre and a diagnosis of myasthenia gravis was confirmed with antibody and electrophysiological tests. A computed tomography scan of his thorax was normal and he was prescribed oral pyridostigmine.

What is myasthenia gravis?

Myasthenia gravis is an autoimmune disorder of neuromuscular transmission characterised by fatigable muscle weakness. The disorder is typically mediated by antibodies against the postsynaptic acetylcholine receptor or by antibodies against muscle specific tyrosine kinase. About 10% of patients with myasthenia gravis have a thymoma.[1] Any muscle group can be affected in myasthenia gravis, but typically patients present with ocular symptoms, namely diplopia and ptosis. Weakness then becomes generalised in about 80% of patients.[2] The most serious complication is myasthenic crisis: acute respiratory failure resulting from myasthenia gravis that requires mechanical ventilation. Myasthenic crisis occurs in about 20% of patients with myasthenia gravis and is a neurological emergency requiring admission to an intensive care unit for respiratory support.[3]

Why is myasthenia gravis missed?

The fluctuating nature of the symptoms and the often subtle findings on clinical examination can make myasthenia gravis difficult to diagnose. In one study, diagnosis was delayed for more than five years in 13% of patients, and 26% of patients had had an inappropriate non-specific investigation before diagnosis.[8] The symptoms of myasthenia gravis are confined to the eye in about 20% of patients with the condition, which can make diagnosis challenging.[2]

Evidence suggests that myasthenia gravis is under-recognised in elderly people, partly because symptoms such as dysphagia, fatigue, and slurred speech can have a broad differential diagnosis in that group.[9] Myasthenia gravis has been reported to have been mistaken for stroke, Parkinson's disease, and motor neurone disease in elderly people.[9] [10] [11] Signs such as ptosis may also be attributed to aponeurotic ("age related") ptosis (so

---

KEY POINTS

- Suspect myasthenia gravis in patients with fluctuating weakness, which initially is typically ocular, although weakness subsequently becomes more generalised in 80% of patients
- If myasthenia gravis is suspected, refer the patient to a neurology centre for investigations, including testing for the presence of antibodies to the acetylcholine receptor and to muscle specific tyrosine kinase, and specific electrophysiological tests
- The patient may still have myasthenia gravis even if the results of serology and electrophysiological investigations are normal; history is key to the diagnosis
- Effective treatment (including acetylcholinesterase inhibitors and steroids) is available for this potentially fatal condition and should not be discontinued abruptly; patients having surgery or experiencing other stresses need close monitoring and possibly changes in treatment to prevent myasthenic crisis

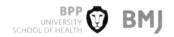

HOW COMMON IS MYASTHENIA GRAVIS?

- The prevalence of myasthenia gravis in the United Kingdom is estimated at about 15 per 100000 population, although this figure has increased over time[4] [5]

- The incidence is bimodal, with a female:male ratio of 2:1 in younger adults and a reversed sex ratio in older people[6]

- Both the incidence and the prevalence of myasthenia gravis in older patients are greater than previously thought[7]

RED FLAGS FOR AN IMMINENT MYASTHENIC CRISIS

- Rapid worsening of primary myasthenic symptoms

- Rapid progression of bulbar symptoms

- Increasing dose of pyridostigmine

- Tachypnoea

- Tachycardia

- Decreased forced vital capacity

- Respiratory infection

---

called because of the stretching of the aponeurosis tendon, which generally occurs in older people).

A diagnosis of myasthenia gravis may be missed in primary and secondary care as some patients may have negative serology results (antibodies) and normal electrophysiology, particularly if they have only ocular myasthenia gravis.[12] Thus a thorough history is central to the diagnosis.

Why does it matter?

Myasthenia gravis is eminently treatable. Untreated patients are at risk of having an acute deterioration of their symptoms and developing myasthenic crisis.

How is it diagnosed?

Clinical

History

The clinical hallmark of myasthenia gravis is fatigable muscle weakness. The history should elicit the pattern and severity of the weakness and any fluctuation of symptoms. Symptoms are typically worse at the end of the day. They may also worsen with heat, infections, surgery, or emotional stress, menstruation, pregnancy, and the post-partum state. Diplopia and ptosis are the most common presenting features of myasthenia gravis, but about 80% of patients will subsequently develop more generalised weakness.[2] Weakness is typically more noticeable in the upper limbs than the lower limbs and is often proximal. Bulbar weakness can manifest as difficulty in chewing or as slurred speech, particularly after a long conversation. Dysphagia, choking, or nasal regurgitation of liquids can herald more severe bulbar weakness. Neck weakness can lead to head drop and neck pain. Respiratory weakness may manifest with exertional dyspnoea or orthopnoea.

Examination

Cranial nerve examination may show ophthalmoplegia or weakness of forced eyelid or mouth closure. Bulbar weakness may be evident if the patient develops dysarthria or nasal speech after prolonged speaking, such as at the end of the consultation or after counting to 50. Fatigability can be elicited by watching for the development of ptosis during sustained upgaze. On examination of the peripheral nervous system, fatigability can be assessed by testing shoulder abduction before and after unilateral repetitive arm movement. There

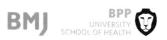

may be obvious weakness of neck flexion or extension, and if diaphragmatic weakness is present, there may be paradoxical abdominal movement during inspiration.

Investigations

Ice test

If the diagnosis of myasthenia gravis is suspected, refer the patient to a neurology unit for further investigations. In patients with ptosis, the ice test is a simple first line test that can be done in the clinic while waiting for other investigations. This distinguishes myasthenia gravis from other causes of ptosis and involves application of crushed ice in a latex glove to the eye for three minutes. In myasthenia gravis this leads to improvement of ptosis and has a sensitivity and specificity of >90%.[13]

Laboratory investigations

The presence of antibodies to the acetylcholine receptor or to muscle specific tyrosine kinase is highly specific. About 85% of patients with generalised myasthenia gravis have antibodies to the acetylcholine receptor, and 40-70% of the rest are positive for antibodies to muscle specific tyrosine kinase.[14] Repeating negative serological tests can be useful because a seroconversion rate of 15% over one year has been reported.[14] Nevertheless, some patients will be persistently seronegative, especially those with only ocular myasthenia gravis.[12]

Levels of muscle specific enzymes such as creatine phosphokinase are usually normal in myasthenia gravis.

Neurophysiology

Routine electrophysiology generally yields normal results in myasthenia gravis, and the diagnosis may be missed if specific electrophysiological tests such as repetitive nerve stimulation and single fibre electromyography are not requested. Repetitive nerve stimulation is specific for myasthenia gravis, but the sensitivity is only 70% and is even lower in disease that is purely ocular.[12] Single fibre electromyography is a selective recording technique that allows identification of action potentials from individual muscle fibres. It is more sensitive (92-100%) than repetitive nerve stimulation for myasthenia gravis but is not specific.[15] Single fibre electromyography is a challenging technique that depends greatly on the skill of the operator and the muscles that are tested as often only affected muscles will show positive results.

Edrophonium test

The edrophonium (Tensilon) test involves intravenous administration of a short acting acetylcholinesterase inhibitor while watching for a transient improvement in muscle strength.[16] The test should be done only when an objective improvement in muscle strength, such as resolution of ptosis, can be shown. Although it has a high sensitivity (95%) for generalised myasthenia gravis, it is now rarely done as it can result in life threatening bradycardia and requires immediate access to resuscitation facilities.

Radiology

Although it does not form part of the diagnostic tests, computed tomography of the thorax is required in all patients in whom myasthenia gravis is diagnosed to exclude the presence of an underlying thymoma.

How is myasthenia gravis managed?

Acetylcholinesterase inhibitors, such as pyridostigmine, provide short lived symptomatic relief and are first line treatment, although they are less useful in myasthenia gravis when patients have antibodies to muscle specific tyrosine kinase.[17] Most patients will require immunomodulatory therapy, started by secondary care.[18] Oral steroids are generally first line immunosuppressive treatment, although side effects limit long term use.[17] High initial doses of

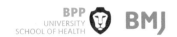

prednisolone can transiently exacerbate weakness, and patients may be admitted to hospital if rapid escalation of treatment is needed.[18] Second line immunosuppressive agents used in myasthenia gravis include azathioprine, mycophenolate mofetil, methotrexate, tacrolimus, and ciclosporin.[17] Rituximab has been used in severe treatment resistant myasthenia gravis.[19] Intravenous immunoglobulin and plasma exchange are reserved for rapidly deteriorating myasthenia gravis and for the treatment of myasthenic crisis.[18]

Thymectomy is a well recognised treatment for myasthenia gravis and should always be performed if a thymoma is suspected.[17 18] Thymectomy is also considered in non-thymomatous generalised myasthenia gravis in patients with antibodies to the acetylcholine receptor who are aged under 50.[18] Thymectomy is not generally carried out in myasthenia gravis when patients have antibodies to muscle specific tyrosine kinase, late onset myasthenia gravis, or purely ocular disease.[18]

Importantly, patients should not abruptly discontinue their treatment for myasthenia gravis. Patients who are dysphagic and cannot take oral medication should be admitted to hospital and other routes of administration, such as nasogastric tubes, should be sought. Moreover, patients who are septicaemic, having surgery, or experiencing some other stress require close monitoring because a change or escalation of their treatment may be needed to prevent myasthenic crisis. Some medications—such as aminoglycoside and quinolone antibiotics, quinine, and intravenous magnesium—are contraindicated in myasthenia gravis as they can impair neuromuscular transmission. A full list of medications that can affect myasthenia gravis is available from the Myasthenia Gravis Foundation of America (www.myasthenia.org).

Contributors: All authors were responsible for the design of the article, drafting it, and revising it critically for intellectual content. All authors approved the final manuscript. JS is the guarantor.

Competing interests: All authors have completed the ICMJE uniform disclosure form at www.icmje.org/coi_disclosure.pdf (available on request from the corresponding author) and declare: no support from any organisation for the submitted work; the Myasthenia Gravis Association UK funds JS's research post; no other relationships or activities that could appear to have influenced the submitted work.

Provenance and peer review: Commissioned; externally peer reviewed.

Patient consent not required (patient anonymised, dead, or hypothetical).

1 Skeie GO, Romi F. Paraneoplastic myasthenia gravis: immunological and clinical aspects. *Eur J Neurol* 2008;15:1029-33.

2 Grob D, Brunner N, Namba T, Pagala M. Lifetime course of myasthenia gravis. *Muscle Nerve* 2008;37:141-9.

3 Jani-Acsadi A, Lisak RP. Myasthenic crisis: guidelines for prevention and treatment. *J Neurol Sci* 2007;15;261:127-33.

4 Carr AS, Cardwell CR, McCarron PO, McConville J. A systematic review of population based epidemiological studies in myasthenia gravis. *BMC Neurol* 2010;10:46.

5 Robertson NP, Deans J, Compston DA. Myasthenia gravis: a population based epidemiological study in Cambridgeshire, England. *J Neurol Neurosurg Psychiatr* 1998;65:492-6.

6 Phillips LH, 2nd. The epidemiology of myasthenia gravis. *Ann N Y Acad Sci* 2003;998:407-12.

7 Aarli JA. Myasthenia gravis in the elderly: is it different? *Ann N Y Acad Sci* 2008;1132:238-43.

8 Beekman R, Kuks JB, Oosterhuis HJ. Myasthenia gravis: diagnosis and follow-up of 100 consecutive patients. *J Neurol* 1997;244:112-8.

9 Libman R, Benson R, Einberg K. Myasthenia mimicking vertebrobasilar stroke. *J Neurol* 2002;249:1512-4.

10 Montero-Odasso M. Dysphonia as first symptom of late-onset myasthenia gravis. *J Gen Intern Med* 2006;21:C4-6.

11 Vincent A, Clover L, Buckley C, Grimley Evans J, Rothwell PM. Evidence of underdiagnosis of myasthenia gravis in older people. *J Neurol Neurosurg Psychiatr* 2003;74:1105-8.

12 Palace J, Vincent A, Beeson D. Myasthenia gravis: diagnostic and management dilemmas. *Curr Opin Neurol* 2001;14:583-9.

13 Reddy AR, Backhouse OC. "Ice-on-eyes", a simple test for myasthenia gravis presenting with ocular symptoms. *Pract Neurol* 2007;7:109-11.

14 Chan KH, Lachance DH, Harper CM, Lennon VA. Frequency of seronegativity in adult-acquired generalized myasthenia gravis. *Muscle Nerve* 2007;36:651-8.

15 AAEM Quality Assurance Committee, American Association of Electrodiagnostic Medicine. Literature review of the usefulness of repetitive nerve stimulation and single fiber EMG in the electrodiagnostic

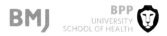

evaluation of patients with suspected myasthenia gravis or Lambert-Eaton myasthenic syndrome. *Muscle Nerve* 2001;24:1239-47.

16 Meriggioli MN, Sanders DB. Advances in the diagnosis of neuromuscular junction disorders. *Am J Phys Med Rehabil* 2005;84:627-38.

17 Gilhus NE, Owe JF, Hoff JM, Romi F, Skeie GO, Aarli JA. Myasthenia gravis: a review of available treatment approaches. *Autoimmune Dis* 2011. doi:10.4061/2011/847393.

18 Skeie GO, Apostolski S, Evoli A, Gilhus NE, Illa I, Harms L, et al. Guidelines for treatment of autoimmune neuromuscular transmission disorders. *Eur J Neurol* 2010;17:893-902.

19 Collongues N, Casez O, Lacour A, Tranchant C, Vermersch P, de Seze J, et al. Rituximab in refractory and non-refractory myasthenia: a retrospective multicenter study. *Muscle Nerve* 2012;46:687-91.

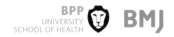

Copper deficiency

S K Chhetri, specialist registrar in neurology[1][2],
R J Mills, consultant neurologist[1],
S Shaunak, consultant neurologist[1],
H C A Emsley, consultant neurologist[1][2]

[1]Department of Neurology, Royal Preston Hospital, Preston PR2 9HT, UK

[2]University of Manchester, Manchester M13 9PL, UK

Correspondence to:
hedley.emsley@manchester.ac.uk

Cite this as: BMJ 2014;348:g3691

DOI: 10.1136/bmj.g3691

www.bmj.com/content/348/bmj.g3691

A 73 year old man with treated pernicious anaemia and partial gastrectomy 30 years earlier consulted his GP with a 12 month history of progressive numbness of his feet and hands. A haematology opinion for normocytic anaemia, neutropenia, and lymphopenia led to an unremarkable bone marrow biopsy. Increasing unsteadiness and falls prompted neurology referral. He was found to have sensory ataxia with clinical, radiological (figure 1), and neurophysiological evidence of myelopathy and peripheral neuropathy. Vitamin B12 level was high, consistent with ongoing replacement. Low serum copper confirmed hypocupraemic myeloneuropathy. Copper replacement achieved resolution of the cytopenia within four weeks, and slow but minimal neurological improvement was seen over more than nine months of follow-up.

What is hypocupraemia?
Copper is an essential trace element that plays a crucial role in the normal functioning of the neurological, haematological, vascular, skeletal, and antioxidant systems.[1][2] Copper is absorbed in the stomach and proximal duodenum, but absorption can be impaired after upper gastrointestinal surgery. Such surgery, although not the sole cause of copper deficiency (hypocupraemia), is increasingly recognised as an important risk factor.[3] Copper deficiency leads to several clinical presentations including cytopenia and profound neurological deficits.[1][2][3][4]

How common is copper deficiency?
Evidence is limited but several reports describe symptomatic copper deficiency.[1][2][3][4][5] In a case series of 136 patients with gastric bypass surgery, 9.6% had hypocupraemia.[6] Two other case series of 64 and 141 bariatric surgery patients respectively reported substantial hypocupraemia in 23% at 6 months and 70% at 3 years,[7] and a progressive reduction in average serum copper concentrations over five years.[8]

Reliable data on the overall population at risk of hypocupraemia from all causes, including bariatric surgery, are not available, but longitudinal collection of data would be valuable.

Why is copper deficiency missed?
Copper deficiency is an under recognised cause of neurological dysfunction and a spectrum of cytopenias.[1] A retrospective review of 40 patients with hypocupraemia found the median interval from initial presentation with neurological or haematological findings to diagnosis of copper deficiency to be 1.1 years (range 10 weeks to 23 years).[2] Misdiagnosis

---

KEY POINTS

- Copper deficiency is an under recognised cause of cytopenias and myeloneuropathy
- Copper deficiency may masquerade as a myelodysplastic syndrome or vitamin B12 deficiency; it might also co-exist with B12 deficiency
- The neurological sequelae of copper deficiency can be debilitating and irreversible, making prompt recognition and treatment essential for successful outcomes
- Clinicians should have a low threshold for measuring serum copper in patients with unexplained and refractory cytopenias or myeloneuropathy, especially in the context of previous upper gastrointestinal tract surgical procedures, excess zinc exposure, or malabsorption

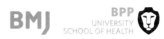

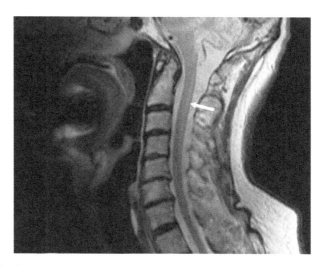

Fig 1 T2 weighted sagittal magnetic resonance image of cervical spine showing increased signal intensity (arrowed) involving dorsal columns of the cervical spinal cord

as a myelodysplastic syndrome might occur, given the similar haematolopathological findings including anaemia, leucopenia, and less commonly, thrombocytopenia.[1][2] This is suggested by a recent retrospective analysis of copper deficiency in Scotland, which found that four out of 16 cases eventually diagnosed with hypocupraemia were initially seen by a haematologist.[1]

The clinical presentation is often clinically and radiologically indistinguishable from subacute combined degeneration (SACD) seen in patients with vitamin B12 deficiency. Confirmation of B12 deficiency in a patient with a clinical presentation resembling SACD might understandably lead to testing for copper deficiency not being undertaken, even though hypocupraemia might be comorbid with B12 deficiency, particularly in patients who have undergone gastric surgery.[4][9]

Moreover, the interval between gastric surgery and the onset of clinical symptoms can be long.[4][5][9] A retrospective review of 55 cases of hypocupraemia found that the interval between upper gastrointestinal surgery and symptom onset ranged from five to 26 years in the bariatric group and 10 to 46 years in the non-bariatric group.[4] Such long intervals might lead to diagnostic delay because a causal association might not be so readily considered, but observations of gradually declining copper levels over years lend clear support to causation.[8]

Why does it matter?
Although copper deficiency is rare, its early identification is essential to minimise its neurological sequelae, which are severely disabling and often irreversible.[1][2][3][4] Copper deficiency can be easily treated and copper supplementation largely prevents further neurological decline, but neurological improvement is variable.[1][2][3][4] A retrospective cohort study in Scotland, which identified 16 patients manifesting clinical sequelae of hypocupraemia (12 with neurological features), found that only 25% of patients show some improvement while 33% might continue to deteriorate with treatment.[1] The haematological effects are relatively easily reversible, with 93% of cytopenias responding to copper replacement and management of the underlying cause.[1]

How is copper deficiency diagnosed?

Clinical features
The diagnosis should be considered in anyone with characteristic neurological or haematological abnormalities (or both), particularly patients with risk factors (box 1). Copper and zinc are competitively absorbed from the gastrointestinal tract; hence zinc excess leads to copper deficiency.[1][4]

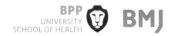

RISK FACTORS FOR COPPER DEFICIENCY[4]

- Upper gastrointestinal tract surgery

- Gastrectomy

- Bariatric surgery

- Small bowel resection or bypass

- Zinc overload

- Zinc supplementation

- Ingestion of zinc containing dental fixatives

- Malabsorption syndromes

Neurological manifestations include myelopathy, myeloneuropathy, and peripheral neuropathy.[1] [4] Patients characteristically present with lower limb paraesthesias and gait disorder with sensory ataxia or spasticity or both.

Investigations

Initial investigations in primary care should include a full blood count and measurement of serum copper. Typical haematological abnormalities are anaemia and leucopenia. Anaemia which might be microcytic, macrocytic, or normocytic, is the commonest cytopenia, followed by leucopenia; thrombocytopenia is infrequent.[1] [2] Laboratory indicators of copper deficiency include low serum copper.[1] [2] [4] Vitamin B12 level should also be tested as B12 deficiency is an important differential diagnosis and may sometimes co-exist with copper deficiency. Zinc levels should also be requested if zinc excess is suspected. American bariatric surgery clinical practice guidelines recommend testing for copper deficiency in post-bariatric surgery patients with anaemia, neutropenia, myeloneuropathy, and impaired wound healing.[10] Specialist referral would generally be pursued for suspected symptomatic hypocupraemia.

Specialist neurological investigations typically include magnetic resonance imaging and neurophysiology. Spinal cord magnetic resonance imaging is abnormal in about 47% of patients with copper deficiency myelopathy and might show increased T2 signal, most commonly in the dorsal midline cervical and thoracic cord.[4] Neurophysiological studies might show axonal sensorimotor polyneuropathy.[4]

How is copper deficiency managed?

Treatment includes management of the underlying cause and copper supplementation. No studies have investigated with the dose, route, duration, or formulation of copper for supplementation. The salts that are commonly used include copper gluconate, copper sulphate, and copper chloride.[4] Copper can be given orally or intravenously. The American Society for Metabolic and Bariatric Surgery Clinical Practice guidelines recommend routine oral copper supplementation (2 mg/d).[10] These guidelines advise intravenous copper (2-4 mg/d) for six days for severe deficiency and subsequent treatment, or treatment of mild to moderate deficiency, with oral copper (3-8 mg/d) until levels normalise.[10] The haematological abnormalities reverse within four to 12 weeks of therapy.[1] Periodic assessment of serum copper is essential to determine adequacy of replacement; however, there are no guidelines to recommend the frequency of monitoring. In patients in whom excess zinc ingestion is the likely cause, discontinuing zinc supplementation might suffice.

We thank Maria Liga (consultant haematologist) and Raza Ansari (general practitioner) for general advice from a haematology and general practice perspective respectively.

Contributors: All authors contributed substantially to the conception and design of this work, its drafting, and/or critical revision for important intellectual content; they all approved the final version and accept accountability for the work.

Having read and understood the BMJ Group policy on declaration of interests, the authors declare that they have no competing interests.

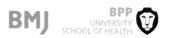

Provenance and peer review: Not commissioned; externally peer reviewed.

Patient consent obtained.

1 Gabreyes AA, Abbasi HN, Forbes KP, McQuaker G, Duncan A, Morrison I. Hypocupremia associated cytopenia and myelopathy: a national retrospective review. *Eur J Haematol* 2013;90:1-9.

2 Halfdanarson TR, Kumar N, Li CY, Phyliky RL, Hogan WJ. Hematological manifestations of copper deficiency: a retrospective review. *Eur. J. Haematol.* 2008;80:523-31.

3 Yarandi SS, Griffith DP, Sharma R, Mohan A, Zhao VM, Ziegler TR. Optic Neuropathy, Myelopathy, Anemia, and Neutropenia Caused by Acquired Copper Deficiency After Gastric Bypass Surgery. *J Clin Gastroenterol* 2014;[Epub ahead of print].

4 Jaiser SR, Winston GP. Copper deficiency myelopathy. *J Neurol* 2010;257:869-81.

5 Robinson SD, Cooper B, Leday TV. Copper deficiency (hypocupremia) and pancytopenia late after gastric bypass surgery. *Proc (Bayl Univ Med Cent)* 2013;26:382-6.

6 Gletsu-Miller N, Broderius M, Frediani JK, Zhao VM, Griffith DP, Davis SS, et al. Incidence and prevalence of copper deficiency following roux-en-y gastric bypass surgery. *Int. J. Obes.* 2012;36:328-35.

7 de Luis DA, Pacheco D, Izaola O, Terroba MC, Cuellar L, Martin T. Clinical results and nutritional consequences of biliopancreatic diversion: three years of follow-up. *Ann Nutr Metab* 2008;53:234-9.

8 Balsa JA, Botella-Carretero JI, Gómez-Martín JM, Peromingo R, Arrieta F, Santiuste C, Zamarrón I, Vázquez C. Copper and zinc serum levels after derivative bariatric surgery: differences between Roux-en-Y Gastric bypass and biliopancreatic diversion. *Obes Surg* 2011;21:744-50.

9 Griffith DP, Liff DA, Ziegler TR, Esper GJ, Winton EF. Acquired copper deficiency: a potentially serious and preventable complication following gastric bypass surgery. *Obesity* 2009;17:827-31.

10 Mechanick JI, Youdim A, Jones DB, Timothy Garvey W, Hurley DL, Molly McMahon M, et al. Clinical practice guidelines for the perioperative nutritional, metabolic, and nonsurgical support of the bariatric surgery patient—2013 update: cosponsored by American Association of Clinical Endocrinologists, the Obesity Society, and American Society for Metabolic and Bariatric Surgery. *Surg Obes Relat Dis* 2013;9:159-91.

Related links

bmj.com/archive

Previous articles in this series
- Bladder cancer in women (BMJ 2014;348:g2171)
- Subdural haematoma in the elderly (BMJ 2014;348:g1682)
- Intestinal malrotation and volvulus in infants and children (BMJ 2013;347:f6949)
- Lisfranc injuries (BMJ 2013;347:f4561)
- Spontaneous oesophageal rupture (BMJ 2013;346:f3095)

More titles in
The BMJ Series

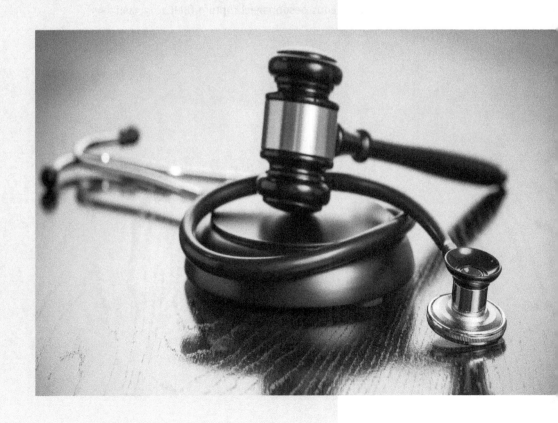

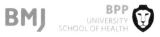
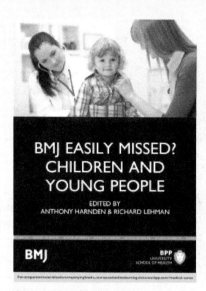
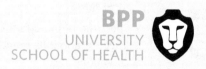

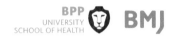
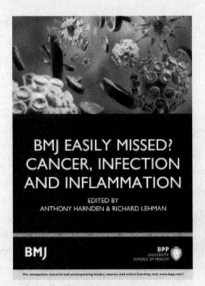
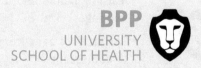

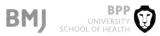
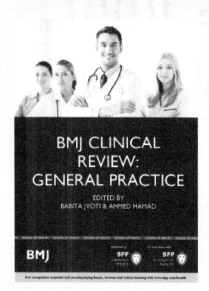
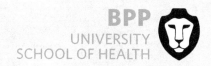

More titles from BPP School of Health

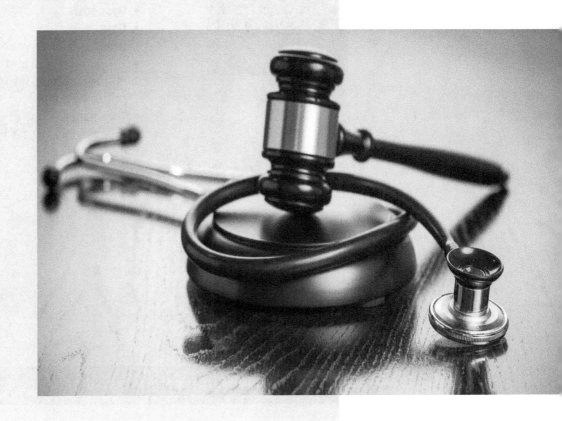

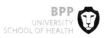

More titles in The Progressing your Medical Career Series

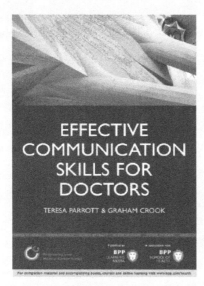

£19.99

September 2011

Paperback

978-1-445379-56-2

Would you like to know how to improve your communication skills? Are you looking for a clearly written book which explores all aspects of effective medical communication?

There is an urgent need to improve doctors' communication skills. Research has shown that poor communication can contribute to patient dissatisfaction, lack of compliance and increased medico-legal problems. Improved communication skills will impact positively on all of these areas.

The last fifteen years have seen unprecedented changes in medicine and the role of doctors. Effective communication skills are vital to these new roles. But communication is not just related to personality. Skills can be learned which can make your communication more effective, and help you to improve your relationships with patients, their families and fellow doctors.

This book shows how to learn those skills and outlines why we all need to communicate more effectively. Healthcare is increasingly a partnership. Change is happening at all levels, from government directives to patient expectations. Communication is a bridge between the wisdom of the past and the vision of the future.

Readers of this book can also gain free access to an online module which upon successful completion can download a certificate for their portfolio of learning/ Revalidation/CPD records.

This easy-to-read guide will help medical students and doctors at all stages of their careers improve their communication within a hospital environment.

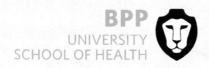

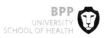

www.bpp.com/medical-series

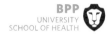

More titles in The Progressing your Medical Career Series

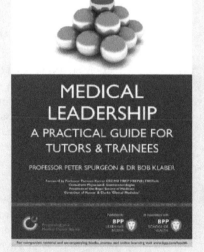

MEDICAL LEADERSHIP

A PRACTICAL GUIDE FOR TUTORS & TRAINEES

PROFESSOR PETER SPURGEON & DR BOB KLABER

£19.99

November 2011

Paperback

978-1-445379-57-9

Are you a doctor or medical student who wishes to acquire and develop your leadership and management skills? Do you recognise the role and influence of strong leadership and management in modern medicine?

Clinical leadership is something in which all doctors should have an important role in terms of driving forward high quality care for their patients. In this up-to-date guide Peter Spurgeon and Robert Klaber take you through the latest leadership and management thinking, and how this links in with the Medical Leadership Competency Framework. As well as influencing undergraduate curricula and some of the concepts underpinning revalidation, this framework forms the basis of the leadership component of the curricula for all medical specialties, so a practical knowledge of it is essential for all doctors in training.

Using case studies and practical exercises to provide a strong work-based emphasis, this practical guide will enable you to build on your existing experiences to develop your leadership and management skills, and to develop strategies and approaches to improving care for your patients.

This book addresses:

- Why strong leadership and management are crucial to delivering high quality care

- The theory and evidence behind the Medical Leadership Competency Framework

- The practical aspects of leadership learning in a wide range of clinical environments (eg handover, EM, ward etc)

- How Consultants and trainers can best facilitate leadership learning for their trainees and students within the clinical work-place

Whether you are a medical student just starting out on your career, or an established doctor wishing to develop yourself as a clinical leader, this practical, easy-to-use guide will give you the techniques and knowledge you require to excel.

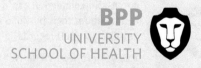

BPP
UNIVERSITY
SCHOOL OF HEALTH

www.bpp.com/medical-series

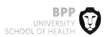

More Titles in The Progressing Your Medical Career Series

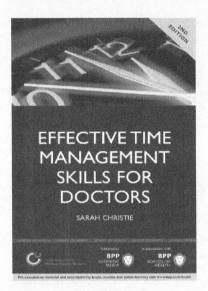

£19.99

January 2012

Paperback

978-1-445390-15-4

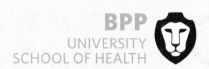
BPP
UNIVERSITY
SCHOOL OF HEALTH

Do you find it difficult to achieve a work-life balance? Would you like to know how you can become more effective with the time you have?

With the introduction of the European Working Time Directive, which will severely limit the hours in the working week, it is more important than ever that doctors improve their personal effectiveness and time management skills. This interactive book will enable you to focus on what activities are needlessly taking up your time and what steps you can take to manage your time better.

By taking the time to read through, complete the exercises and follow the advice contained within this book you will begin to:

- Understand where your time is being needlessly wasted

- Discover how to be more assertive and learn how to say 'No'

- Set yourself priorities and stick to them

- Learn how to complete tasks more efficiently

- Plan better so you can spend more time doing the things you enjoy

In recent years, with the introduction of the NHS Plan and Lord Darzi's commitment to improve the quality of healthcare provision, there is a need for doctors to become more effective within their working environment. This book will offer you the chance to regain some clarity on how you actually spend your time and give you the impetus to ensure you achieve the tasks and goals which are important to you.

www.bpp.com/medical-series

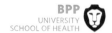

More titles in The Essential Clinical Handbook Series

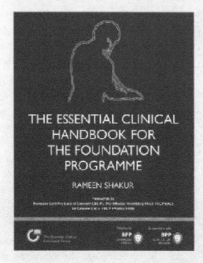

THE ESSENTIAL CLINICAL HANDBOOK FOR THE FOUNDATION PROGRAMME

RAMEEN SHAKUR

£24.99

October 2011

Paperback

978-1-445381-63-3

Unsure of what clinical competencies you must gain to successfully complete the Foundation Programme? Unclear on how to ensure your ePortfolio is complete to enable your progression to ST training?

This up-to-date clinical handbook is aimed at current foundation doctors and clinical medical students and provides a comprehensive companion to help you in the day-to-day management of patients on the ward. Together with this it is the first handbook to also outline clearly how to gain the core clinical competencies required for successful completion of the Foundation Programme. Written by doctors for doctors this comprehensive handbook explains how to successfully manage all of the common cases you will face during the Foundation Programme and:

- Introduces the Foundation Programme and what is expected of a new doctor especially with the introduction of Modernising Medical Careers

- Illustrates clearly the best way to manage, step-by-step, over 150 commonly encountered clinical diseases, including NICE guidelines to ensure a gold standard of clinical care is achieved

- Describes how to successfully gain the core clinical competencies within Medicine and Surgery including an extensive list of differentials and conditions explained

- Explores the various radiology images you will encounter and how to interpret them

- Tells you how to succeed in the assessment methods used including DOP's, Mini-CEX's and CBD's

- Has step by step diagrammatic guide to doing common clinical procedures competently and safely

- Outlines how to ensure your ePortfolio is maintained properly to ensure successful completion of the Foundation Programme

- Provides tips and advice on how to start preparing now to ensure you are fully prepared and have the competitive edge for your CMT/ST application

The introduction of the e-Portfolio as part of the Foundation Programme has paved the way for foundation doctors to take charge of their own learning and portfolio. Through following the expert guidance laid down in this handbook you will give yourself the best possible chance of progressing successfully through to CMT/ST training.

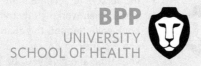

BPP
UNIVERSITY
SCHOOL OF HEALTH

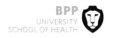

More titles in The Essential Clinical Handbook Series

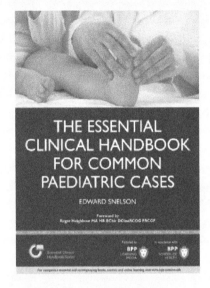

THE ESSENTIAL
CLINICAL HANDBOOK
FOR COMMON
PAEDIATRIC CASES

EDWARD SNELSON

£24.99

September 2011

Paperback

978-1-445379-60-9

Not sure what to do when faced with a crying baby and demanding parent on the ward? Would you like a definitive guide on how to manage commonly encountered paediatric cases?

This clear and concise clinical handbook has been written to help healthcare professionals approach the initial assessment and management of paediatric cases commonly encountered by Junior Doctors, GPs, GP Specialty Trainee's and allied healthcare professionals. The children who make paediatrics so fun, can also make it more than a little daunting for even the most confident person. This insightful guide has been written based on the author's extensive experience within both a General Practice and hospital setting.

Intended as a practical guide to common paediatric problems it will increase confidence and satisfaction in managing these conditions. Each chapter provides a clear structure for investigating potential paediatric illnesses including clinical and non-clinical advice covering: background, how to assess, pitfalls to avoid, FAQs and what to tell parents. This helpful guide provides:

- A problem/symptom based approach to common paediatric conditions

- An essential guide for any doctor assessing children on the front line

- Provides easy-to-follow and step-by-step guidance on how to approach different paediatric conditions

- Useful both as a textbook and a quick reference guide when needed on the ward

This engaging and easy to use guide will provide you with the knowledge, skills and confidence required to effectively diagnose and manage commonly encountered paediatric cases both within a primary and secondary care setting.

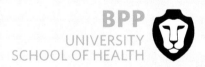

BPP
UNIVERSITY
SCHOOL OF HEALTH

www.bpp.com/medical-series

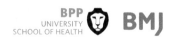